A Doctor's Cure for Medical Myths:
50 Teaspoons of Truth to Remedy Medical Misinformation

Dominic Gaziano, M.D.

First Printing, 2019

Distributed by Bublish, Inc.

ISBN: 978-1-950282-47-0

INTRODUCTION

"THE TRUTH WILL SET YOU FREE," but in my opinion the practice of discerning truth will give you flight.

I'm Dominic Gaziano, M.D., a primary care physician who practices medicine in inner-city Chicago. I live on the front lines of medicine, and I've seen it all. Every day, I see the disturbing consequences suffered by those who believe the many medical myths that "inform" people's medical and health decisions these days. Never, in the history of medicine, has there been so much misinformation so readily available. In a recent article about misinformation on the web, The New York Times starts," Fake news threatens our democracy, Fake medical news threatens our lives." Dr. G here concurs and is writing this book to do something about this.

One of the saddest stories I've heard came from one of my colleagues, an infectious disease doctor here in Chicago. I ran into her in the doctor's lounge at the hospital one day. She looked upset and shared the story of her 26-year-old female patient who routinely refused to get a flu shot. Unfortunately, the patient contracted a very severe case of Influenza A. Despite aggressive treatment in an Intensive Care Unit at one of our top local hospitals, the young woman passed away of a rare complication of the flu, a heart infection called myocarditis. This was a needless death of an otherwise healthy young woman. It is a devastating story that sadly is becoming more common. According to the Center for Disease Control, some 80,000 people in the US died of flu during the winter of 2017. It was the highest death toll in 40 years. Most likely, the death of this young woman in the prime of her life may have been prevented with a simple flu vaccine. Many other flu deaths could also have been prevented.

I see a lot of "vaccine hesitancy" among my patients. They've heard or read about side effects, like you can get the flu from the flu vaccine (a myth I address in this book). The decision not to vaccinate is a dangerous gamble, and one that not only impacts individuals, but families and whole communities as well. Consider the recent outbreaks of measles in New York, Washington, Texas, Illinois, and California. These outbreaks occurred because too many individuals decided to opt out of their vaccination regime, making a whole population vulnerable to the resurgence of a deadly, but once-eradicated disease, like measles.

With medical misinformation, the stakes are high. It's why I decided to write this book. What's the "cure" for medical misinformation? Facts! Cold...Hard...Facts. Inside these pages, I will debunk 50 of the most common medical myths by providing peer-reviewed research and well-documented facts that support the truth. I call these my "50 teaspoons of truth to remedy medical misinformation." I hope you will take the time to read about these myths. I hope you will share and discuss the facts in this book with your family and friends. I hope the next time you hear someone spout off a medical myth—which could possibly put their life at risk—you can calmly inform them of the facts you find in these pages.

As I said, the stakes are high. It's very difficult to reverse popular beliefs once they've found an audience. *A Doctor's Cure for Medical Myths: 50 Teaspoons of Truth to Remedy Medical Misinformation* is my contribution to the discussion. It's my mission to put the facts front and center. Being healthy is a choice, but it should be a well-informed choice. You need facts, not fiction to make the right decisions about your health and well-being. This book provides facts and will hopefully help debunk some of the medical misinformation that threatens the health and well-being of our population.

I wish you well on your journey of truth, health and happiness!

Cheers,
Dr. G

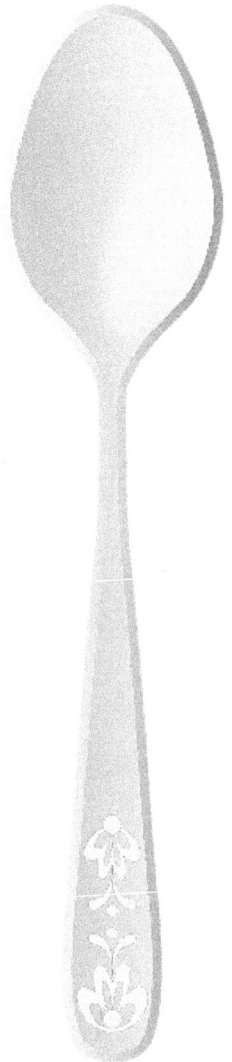

TABLE OF CONTENTS

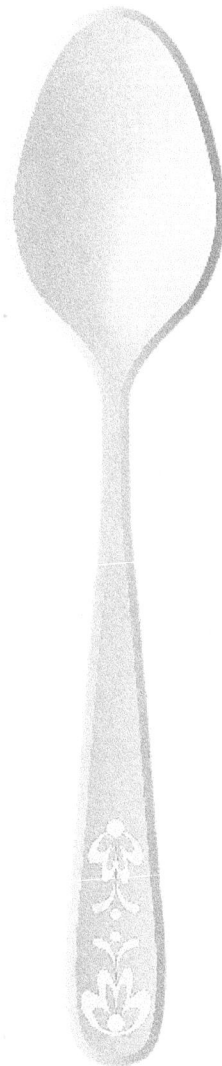

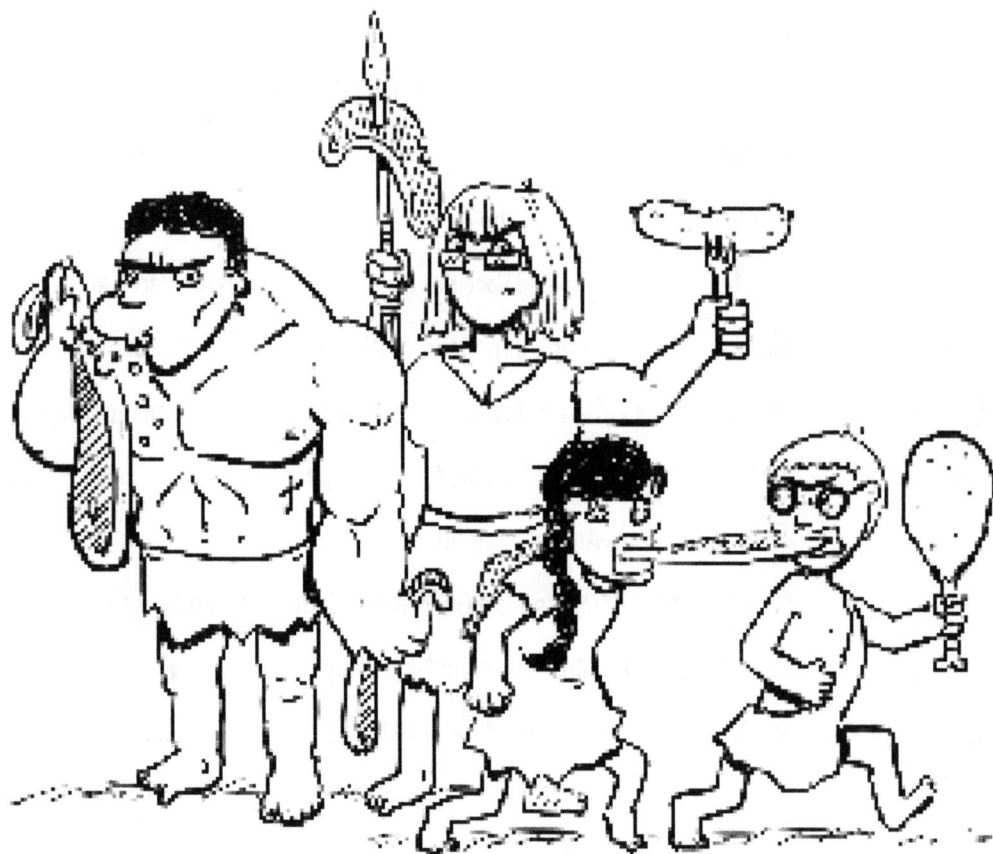

"We Love Meat!"

MYTH Keto Diets Are a Healthy Way to Lose Weight

TRUTH Keto Diets Have Troubling Side Effects.

DIETERS HAVE A MIND-BOGGLING NUMBER of choices these days–everything from The Cabbage Soup Diet to The Beer Diet (not kidding) to the Keto Diet, and so many more. The Ketogenic Diet (aka Keto Diet) restricts the number of carbohydrates consumed in a day, typically to 30 to 50 grams. To replace those calories, the Keto Diet encourages consumption of large amounts of protein and fats. The goal is to move your body into a state of ketosis, a normal metabolic process in which the body burns stored fats because it doesn't have enough glucose (energy created by carbohydrates) to burn. In other words, the Keto Diet compels your body to burn unwanted fat by forcing it to rely on that fat for basic energy.

But here's the dark side of this diet: many health experts now say a high-fat Keto Diet can actually shorten your life. Some nutritionists say this diet can be used for a brief period of time but is not safe for the long-term. On these low-carb diets, you can end up with significant vitamin and mineral deficiencies because you did not get the vitamins and minerals you needed from the fruits and vegetables you were told not to eat because they were high in carbohydrates.

What surprises me as a physician is that ketosis has been known for a long time in the medical and diet world. Most dietitians and weight-loss experts understand that the state of ketosis can lead to weight loss, but they only prescribe it temporarily. They understand that ketosis is not meant to be a perpetual state. Unfortunately, when dieters are not supervised by their doctors, they can get into trouble by following the restrictions of the Keto Diet for too long.

PS. Another side-effect of this diet is that you can end up with perpetual bad breath, which ketosis can cause. Does that sound attractive to you?

"Enjoy the Bread Blues!"

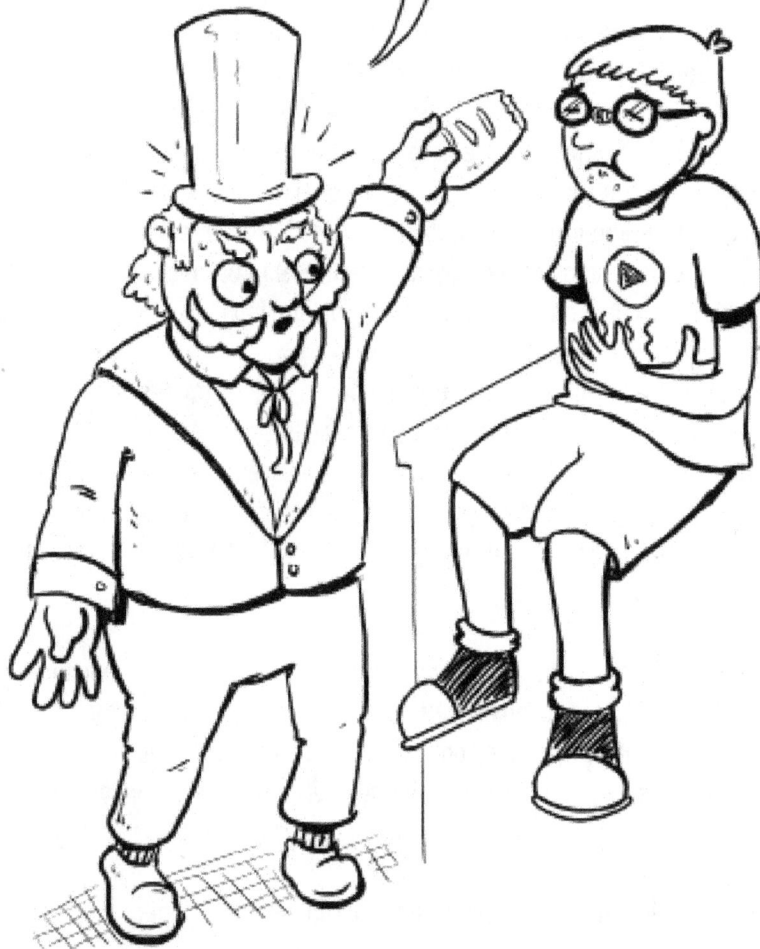

2

MYTH Gluten is Bad for You

TRUTH Not Everyone Should Avoid Gluten

YOU CAN'T GO TO A grocery store these days without seeing hundreds of products that are labeled "Gluten-Free." No one even mentioned gluten 15 years ago–now it's a hot topic. But is gluten bad for you? Let's dive in.

Gluten is a "gluey" protein naturally found in many whole grains like wheat and barley. It helps breads and baked goods hold their shape. In the United States alone, more than 3 million people have sworn off gluten for "health" reasons. The truth is, most people can eat gluten with no side effects. In fact, those who avoid gluten without medical cause may be missing out on the health benefits of nutritional whole grains. Many studies have linked whole grain consumption with improved health outcomes.

The reality is that less than one percent of the US population is allergic to gluten. These individuals suffer from Celiac Disease, which can be life threatening. A second group of people may suffer from some type of gluten sensitivity, but researchers disagree on this. According to a May 23, 2018 article in *Science* magazine, "Some researchers are convinced that many patients have an immune reaction to gluten or another substance in wheat–a nebulous illness sometimes called non-celiac gluten sensitivity (NCGS). Others believe most patients are actually reacting to an excess of poorly absorbed carbohydrates present in wheat and many other foods. Those carbohydrates–called FODMAPs, for fermentable oligosaccharides, disaccharides, monosaccharides, and polyols–can cause bloating when they ferment in the gut. If FODMAPs are the primary culprit, thousands of people may be on gluten-free diets with the support of their doctors and dietitians but without good reason."

Many patients in my practice boast that they are on a gluten-free diet, as if it's something that will improve their health. They are proud to be gluten-free. When I mention that scientific research shows that gluten isn't bad for you unless you have specific medical conditions, they just shrug off the facts. Ironically, my patients who suffer from Celiac Disease and can't consume any gluten, wish they could. For this one percent, gluten is definitely off limits. But for most people, pasta and bread lovers around the world, I say "Manga! Manga!"

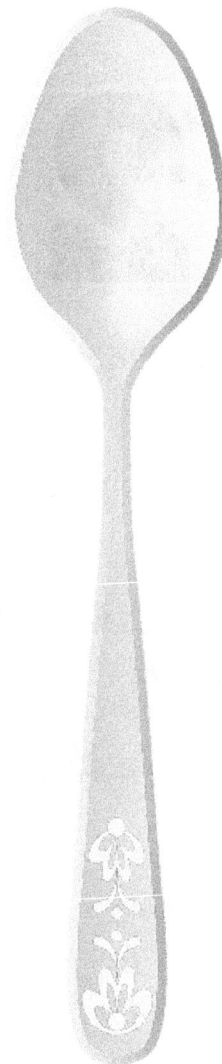

"Many studies have linked whole grain consumption with improved health outcomes."

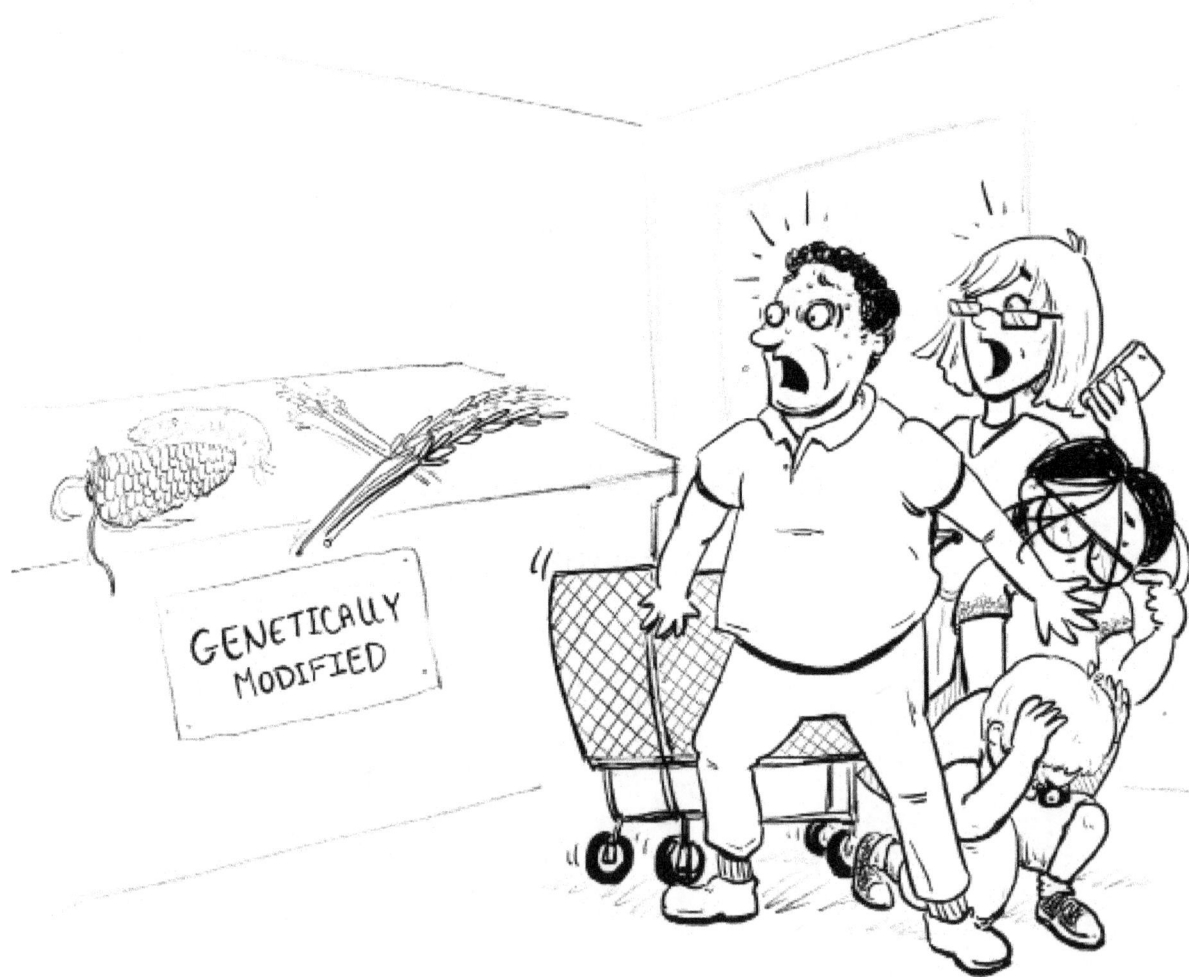

"Run! It's Mutant Corn!"

3

MYTH GMO Foods Are Bad for You
TRUTH There Is Not Strong Evidence that GMO Foods Are Unsafe

GENETICALLY MODIFIED ORGANISMS (GMOs) ARE PLANTS and animals whose DNA has been altered in a laboratory. A review by the National Academy of Sciences looked at more than 20 years of research and 900 studies and did not find any evidence that GMOs pose a hazard to human health. Yet, this hasn't silenced debate about their safety.

According to an article in *Scientific American*, "The Truth about Genetically Modified Food," the benefits outweigh the potential for theoretical risks. "The vast majority of the research on genetically modified crops suggests that they are safe to eat and that they have the potential to feed millions of people worldwide who currently go hungry." The concern among a small number of scientists is that since the first GMO crops hit the market in the 1990s, we haven't had enough time to understand generationally how the introduction of a gene into a different genome can impact it down the road.

There are many important benefits provided by genetically modified crops and the foods made with them. The *Scientific American* article goes on to state that "The bulk of the science on GM safety points in one direction. Take it from David Zilberman, a UC Berkeley agricultural and environmental economist and one of the few researchers considered credible by both agricultural chemical companies and their critics. He argues that the benefits of GM crops greatly outweigh the health risks, which so far remain theoretical. The use of GM crops "has lowered the price of food," Zilberman says. "It has increased farmer safety by allowing them to use less pesticide. Yes, less pesticide, this is a good thing. It has raised the output of corn, cotton and soy by 20 to 30 percent, allowing some people to survive who would not have without it. If it were more widely adopted around the world, the price [of food] would go lower, and fewer people would die of hunger."

Concern about food safety is important. We should never stop questioning the methods used to produce the foods we consume. I do, however, believe that concerns about genetically modified foods are misplaced and that the real advantages of genetic modification far outweigh any disadvantages.

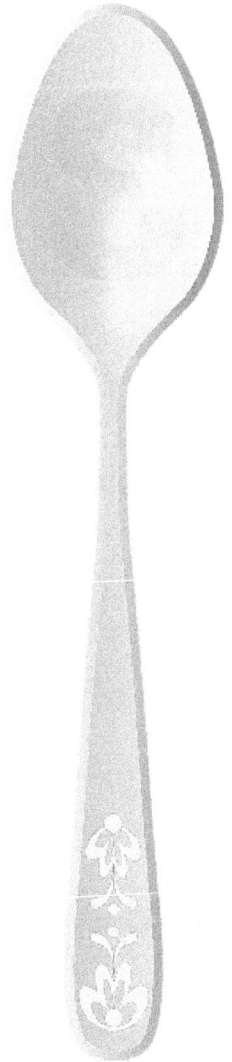

"The real advantages of genetic modification far outweigh any disadvantages."

"If Only Your Heart Could Talk."

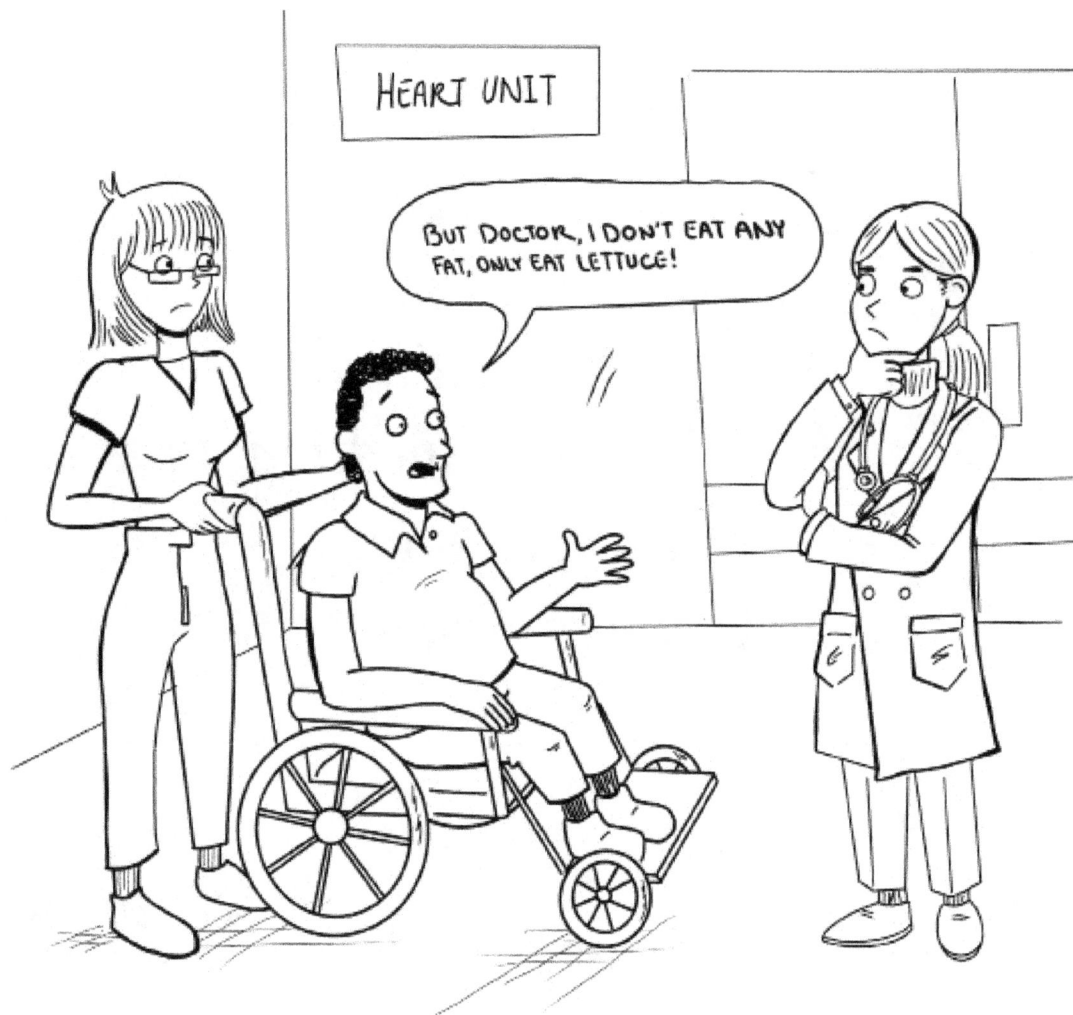

4

MYTH Cholesterol Can Be Controlled by Diet Alone
TRUTH Some People Need to Take Medication for High Cholesterol

IT WOULD BE NICE IF you could control your cholesterol by diet alone, but unfortunately, it isn't always possible. Cholesterol is complicated. Not only is there "good" cholesterol (HDL) and "bad cholesterol" (LDL), there are those nasty triglycerides.

We all produce lipids (cholesterol and triglycerides) naturally every day, but some of us produce higher levels and process them less efficiently. It's genetic. We can thank our parents for the genes they gave us. Some of us have genes that predispose us to hyperlimedemia, which causes an abnormally high concentration of fats or lipids in the blood. This is what high LDL and high triglyceride levels reflect. If you're not genetically prone to "high fat" in your blood, you can typically keep your blood-lipid levels within an acceptable range through diet and exercise. By the way, the exercise part is crucial!

The Pritikin diet, the Ornish diet and the Mediterranean diet all have good numbers for lowering your cholesterol. Reducing your saturated fats, eating foods rich in omega-3 fatty acids like salmon, increasing soluble fiber in food such as oatmeal, and adding more whey protein will decrease your cholesterol. It has been found that these diets had to be strictly followed in order for the person to have significant results. Yes, you may be able to lower your levels somewhere between 10 and 20 percent. However, if you have an LDL level of 180 and your goal is 100, diet and exercise alone cannot get you to your goal.

If you can't get your blood-lipid levels where they need to be through diet and exercise, you should seriously consider a prescription medication such as a statin, which can help your body lower its cholesterol burden. High levels of LDL in the bloodstream, usually over 120, can't typically be lowered through diet and exercise alone. Statins have been proven to be very effective at lowering cholesterol anywhere from 10 to 55 percent. Yet, when I prescribe lipid medications to my patients, many never start taking them. They fear the potential side effects like muscle aches, headaches, and difficulty sleeping—but these are rare. Most of my patients prefer to try to keep their cholesterol levels under control through diet and exercise alone. In my opinion, they are doing their bodies a terrible disservice by ignoring the clear long-term health benefits these drugs provide. Like all medications, lipid-lowering statins can cause side effects. However, studies show that, in certain people, statins can reduce the risk of heart attack and stroke by 25 to 35 percent. Those numbers are even more impressive for recurrent strokes or heart attacks—about 40 percent. Those are impressive numbers and shouldn't be ignored. If you suffer from high cholesterol, I ask you to weigh the risks and benefits fairly. If you are a patient at risk for a heart attack or stroke, please seriously consider the important role these life-saving medications can play in your health-care regime.

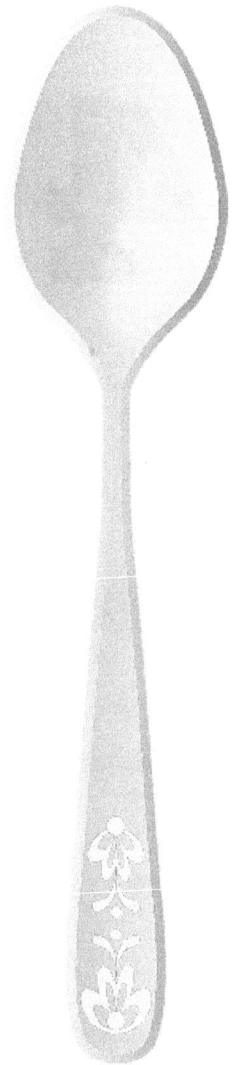

"They are doing their bodies a terrible disservice by ignoring the clear long-term health benefits these drugs provide."

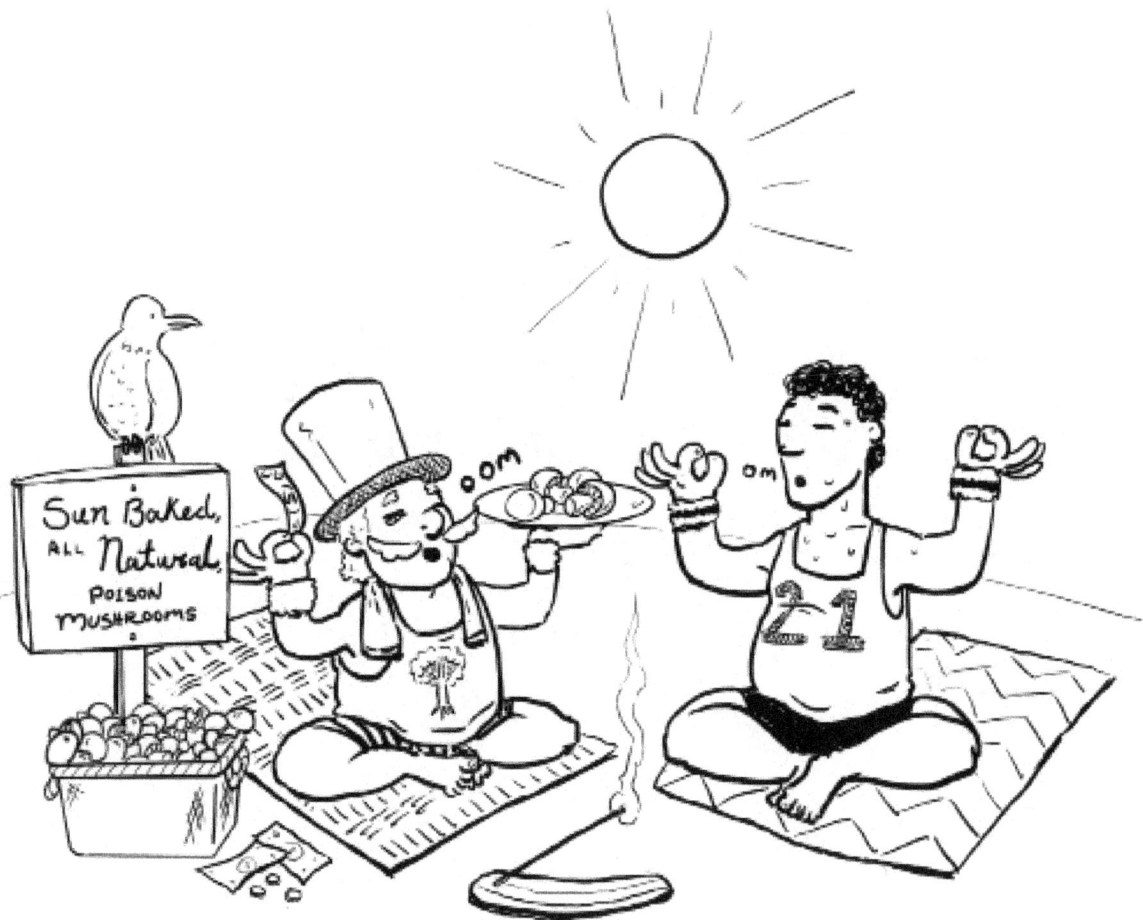

"True Health Nuts"

5

MYTH Foods Labeled "All Natural" Are Always Better for You
TRUTH Food Labels Don't Tell the Whole Story

FOOD LABELING IN THE UNITED STATES is a tricky business. While knowing how many calories a food product contains or how much protein it has can be useful in making decisions at the grocery store, a growing number of food labels are crafted by marketers, not nutritionists. Walk down any food aisle these days and you'll see claims of "Sugar Free," "Organic," "Non-GMO," "Hormone Free," "Free Range," and more. They indicate a product's attributes, but not necessarily its nutritional value. "All Natural" falls into this category.

According to a 2018 article in *The Globe and Mail* written by Toronto-based dietitian Leslie Beck, "The term 'natural' can be misleading to consumers, many of whom assume it to mean 'healthier' or 'more nutritious.' ...A claim of 'natural ingredients' doesn't speak to the healthfulness of a food product. While 'all natural' almond butter is nutritious, 'all natural' licorice, packed with added sugar, certainly is not....Don't assume, also, that foods labeled natural will be free of pesticide, hormone and antibiotic residues....Ground meat that comes from conventionally raised beef cattle will contain hormone and antibiotic residues even though it's a natural food."

In plain terms, just because something is labeled "All Natural" does not guarantee that it has nutritional benefits or is free of questionable ingredients. As a practicing general internal medicine physician and wellness practitioner for the last 20 years, I have heard scores of pitches from nutrition reps who pitch me "all natural" nutraceutical products. When I ask them to show me the science, many of them have nothing to support their pitch. They do not have anything superior to what you can get in the produce section or at a farmers market, so why not just go there and save some money. "All natural" and "natural" products can still contain pesticides, hormonal residues and artificial ingredients.

In general, yes, it's better to eat natural foods rather than processed or ultra processed foods. Everyone knows that junk food and fast food are bad for you, but processed cheese and processed meats are also unhealthy. Is eating an entire bag of "natural" potato chips going to improve your health? I think you know the answer. Just because something is natural, doesn't guarantee that it's good for you. Many foods found in nature can kill you. Consider the beautiful water hemlock plant. It can cause seizures. It can be fatal if ingested. The beautiful, white Amanita mushroom is called the "death cap" because one bite can kill you. Yes, those are extremes, but my point is: Labels don't tell the whole story about health. More often than not, they are "marketing speak" rather than reliable nutritional data.

If your goal is to buy food that has nutritional value for optimal health, you'll need to look beyond the labels and learn more about what makes up a balanced diet and how to source the best foods to support that diet.

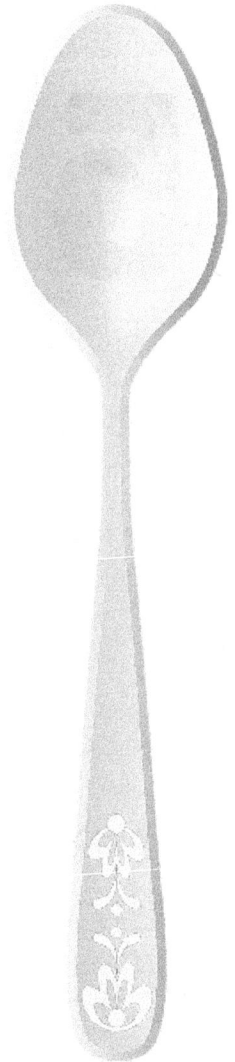

"Just because something is labeled 'all natural' does not guarantee it has nutritional benefits."

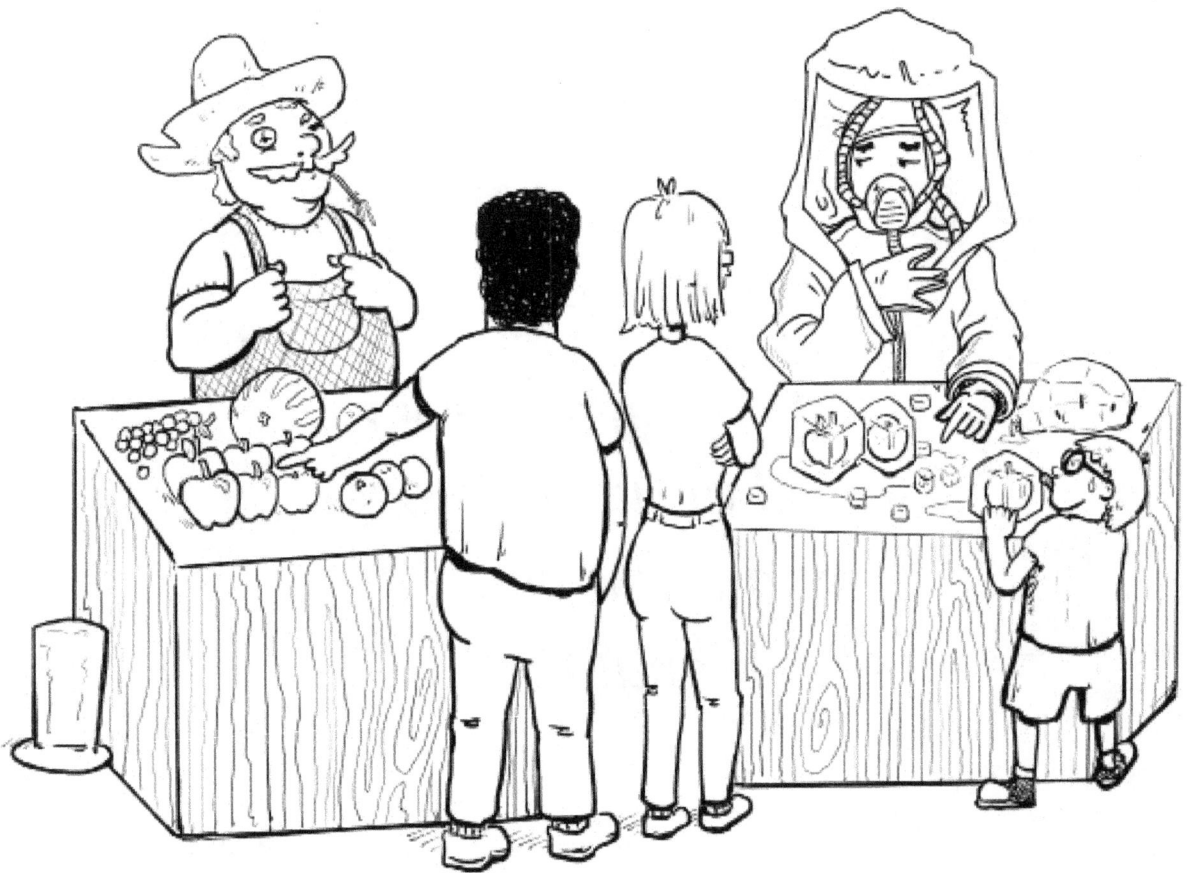

"Ice...Ice....No Way, Baby!"

6

TRUTH Today, Fresh Fruits and Vegetables Are Not More Nutritional than Frozen

IN OLDEN DAYS, PEOPLE HARVESTED the food they ate directly from the land. They milked their cows, picked fresh berries and gathered whole grains. The taste and nutritional value of these foods was unsurpassed, and for those lucky enough to still live this lifestyle, they still are.

Today, however, "fresh" foods often travel for many days before reaching local supermarkets, and ultimately consumers. Today, more people live in cities than on farms. If you can still grow and harvest your own food, by all means, enjoy the benefits. If, however, you live a more average American lifestyle and growing your own fruits and vegetables is difficult, well, I have good news for you. According to a 2015 study by The University of California (UC), "Overall, the vitamin content of the frozen commodities was comparable to and occasionally higher than that of their fresh counterparts."

Yes, you read that right, "occasionally higher." How could this be? Because good old human ingenuity led to "quick frozen" and other technologies that preserve vitamins and minerals during the freezing process. In fact, as the UC study revealed, "Vitamin C was higher in frozen corn, green beans and blueberries than in their fresh equivalents. There was more riboflavin (a B vitamin) in frozen rather than fresh broccoli, though fresh peas had more than frozen ones."

Many of my patients aspire to live healthy lives. However, they work long hours and juggle multiple responsibilities. Finding time to grow their own food or visit the local Farmers' Market isn't always feasible. They need nutritious foods "on demand." Frozen food provides a healthy and convenient solution. Frozen foods are often cheaper than their "fresh" counterparts, too, and are readily available any season of the year.

Try to eat fresh fruits and vegetables whenever you can. But if you're feeling guilty about eating their frozen counterparts, there's no need. That frozen bag of broccoli or peaches will give you the nutrition you need.

Here's a time-saving tip for you: If you can't go to the grocery store weekly, buy a combination of fresh and frozen produce. Eat the fresh fruits and vegetables first and then reach for the frozen, so you do not have to go the grocery store as much. You'll get the nutrition you need without the stress.

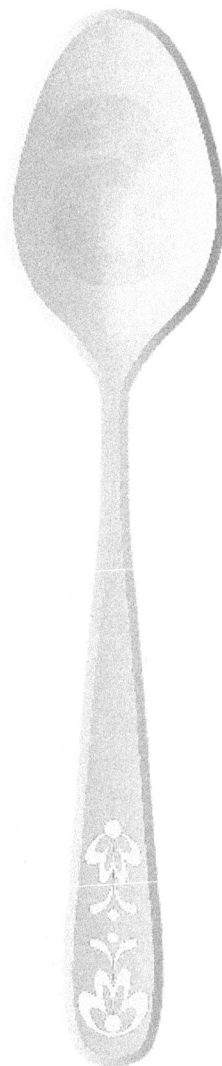

"Overall, the vitamin content of frozen commodities was comparable to and occasional higher than that of their fresh counterparts."

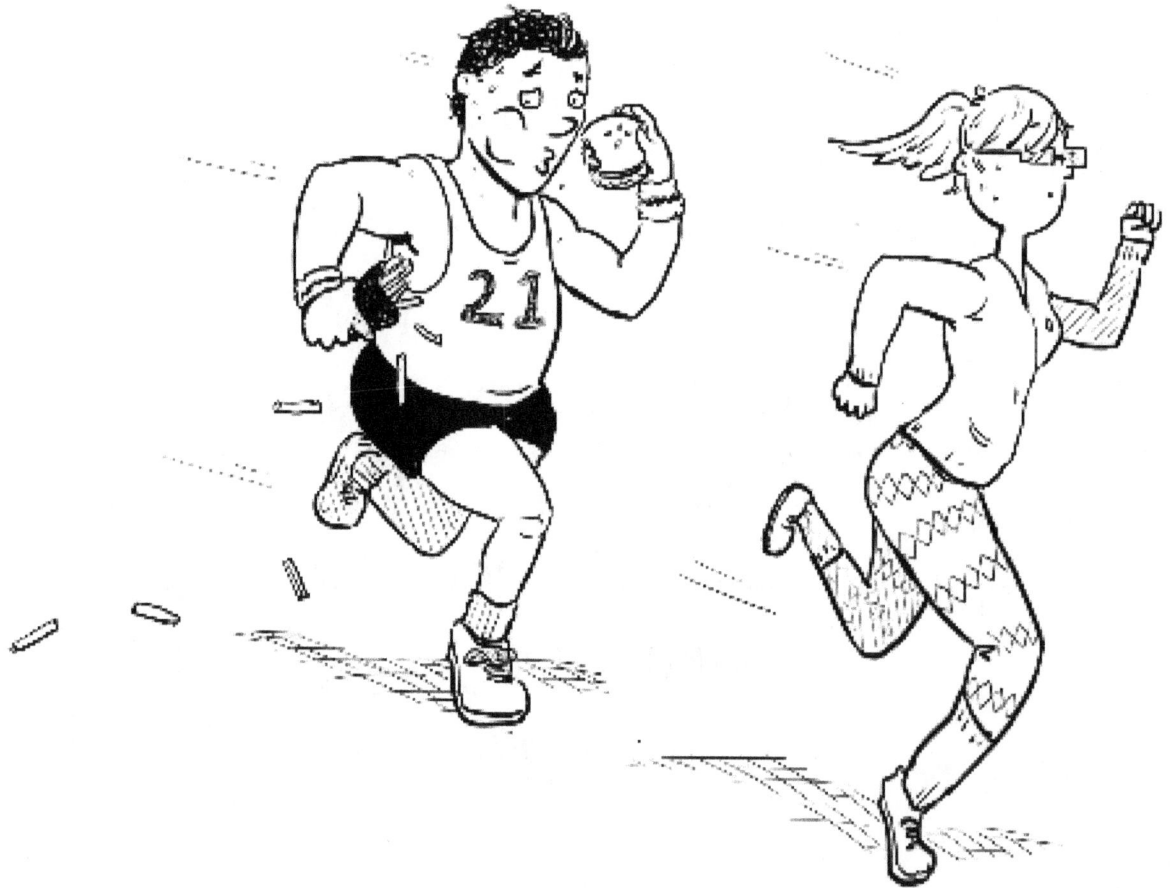

"We're Really in Calorie Burn Mode Now!"

7

MYTH Intense Workouts Guarantee Weight Loss and Health

TRUTH Optimal Health and Weight Loss Require Regular Exercise AND a Balanced Diet

I'VE HEARD MY PATIENTS SAY IT. "Doc, I ate a deep-dish pizza Saturday night, but I ran an hour after to burn it off, so I'm still on track to lose that extra weight we talked about." No, you're not!

If you want to reach your perfect weight and live a healthy life, you'll need to exercise regularly *and* eat a balanced diet. Food not only provides the fuel we need to exercise effectively and efficiently; research shows us that diet plays a major role in losing and keeping off unwanted weight. Certain foods may even have an impact on our appetite and assist in weight loss. More importantly, there is plenty of scientific evidence indicating that daily, moderate exercise combined with a healthy, balanced diet has numerous life-long health benefits.

Amid the many controversial "fad" diets promoted today–some of which can actually be dangerous–there are sustainable and healthy lifestyle diets that focus on optimal health and weight, rather than quick weight loss. I recommend the highly researched and time-tested Mediterranean-lifestyle diet, with its emphasis on plant-based foods (such as fruits and vegetables, whole grains, legumes and nuts). The diet also suggests eating plenty of healthy fats such as olive oil, and cooking with herbs and spices. If you follow this diet, you'll limit your consumption of red meat and have fish and poultry at least twice a week. This lifestyle diet also encourages people to share their meals with family and friends in a social atmosphere. Moderate daily exercise is also suggested. It's all about balance.

The Mayo Clinic writes that "a meta-analysis of more than 1.5 million healthy adults demonstrated that following a Mediterranean diet was associated with a reduced risk of cardiovascular mortality as well as overall mortality. The Mediterranean diet is also associated with a reduced incidence of cancer, and Parkinson's and Alzheimer's diseases. Women who eat a Mediterranean diet supplemented with extra-virgin olive oil and mixed nuts may have a reduced risk of breast cancer."

The next time you're offered a chocolate sundae and think you can just run it off...think again. Make better choices about the food you eat and exercise regularly. You'll feel better, achieve more sustainable results, *and* live a healthier life.

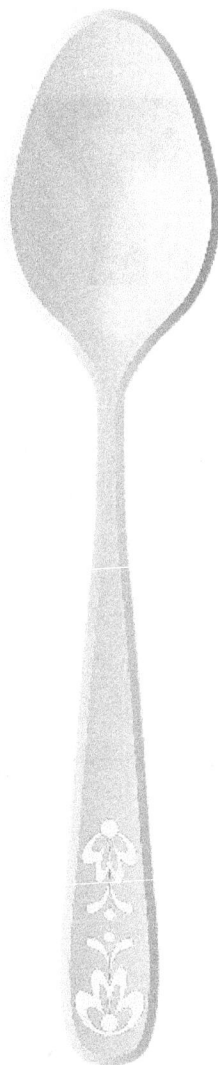

"The next time you're offered a chocolate sundae and think you can just run it off... think again."

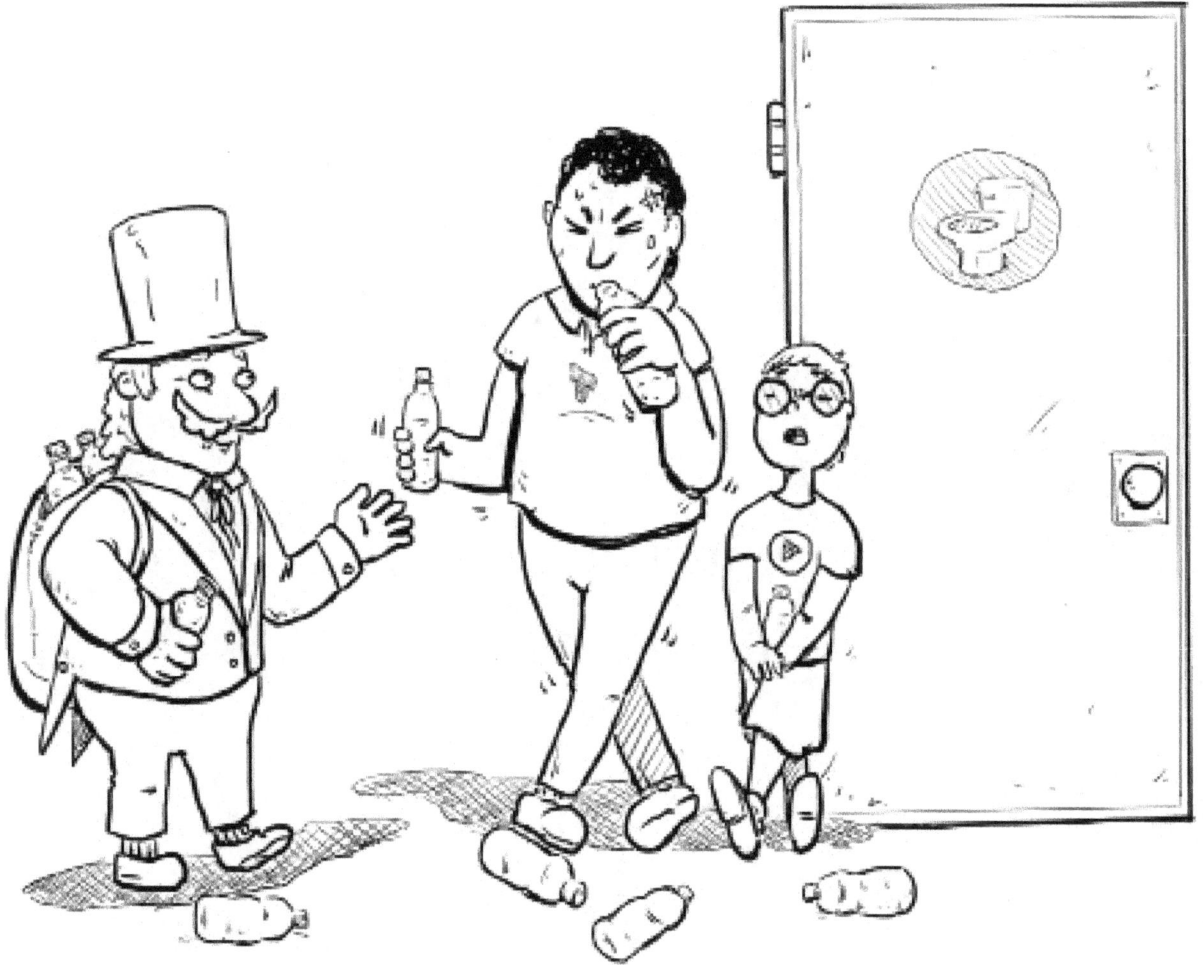

"Welcome to Hydration Nation!"

MYTH You Must Drink 8 Glasses of Water a Day to Be Healthy

TRUTH Everyone's Water Needs Are Different

THIS IS ONE OF THOSE "ONE-SIZE-FITS-ALL" myths, and it's a gross oversimplification of the truth. There's absolutely no scientific proof that the so-called "8 by 8" formula (eight ounces of water, eight times a day) is valid. No one knows exactly where this myth started. Some blame the bottled water industry; others believe a 1945 recommendation by the US National Research Council (NRC) shaped the myth.

No matter where the myth originated, the reality is that most people don't need to consciously think about water intake at all, because the thirst mechanism in the brain is very effective at giving us a heads-up that it's time to hydrate. The health benefits of water are well known. Water helps our bodies get rid of waste through urination, perspiration and bowel movements. It keeps our temperature normal, lubricates our joints, and protects sensitive tissue. But individual water needs depend on a variety of factors—where you live, how often you exercise, your overall health, and whether you are pregnant or breastfeeding, just to name a few.

We actually get 20 percent of our daily intake of water from the food we eat. Cucumbers, for example, are 96.7 percent water. Iceberg lettuce is 95.6 percent water and celery is 95.4 percent water. Tomatoes, radishes, green peppers, watermelon, spinach, strawberries, broccoli, and cauliflower are other examples of foods with a water content level above 90 percent. Chances are, if you're a healthy eater, you're getting a good portion of your daily water intake from the fruits and vegetables you eat as part of a healthy diet.

If you feel hydrated and your urine is colorless or light yellow, most likely you are adequately hydrated. There's no need to guzzle water bottle after water bottle to meet some arbitrary intake level. It's about balance and listening to your body.

Did you know it is actually possible to drink too much water? Though rare, a condition called hyponatremia, also known as water intoxication, can be dangerous. Drinking an extreme amount of water in a short time can actually be fatal. Drinking too much water too fast can cause the level of salt, or sodium, in your blood to drop too low. It can put a strain on your kidneys and ultimately your brain.

Water consumption is very important for health, but before you believe the "one size fits all" myth that you need 8 glasses of water a day, listen to your body. Most of the time, it will tell you the truth.

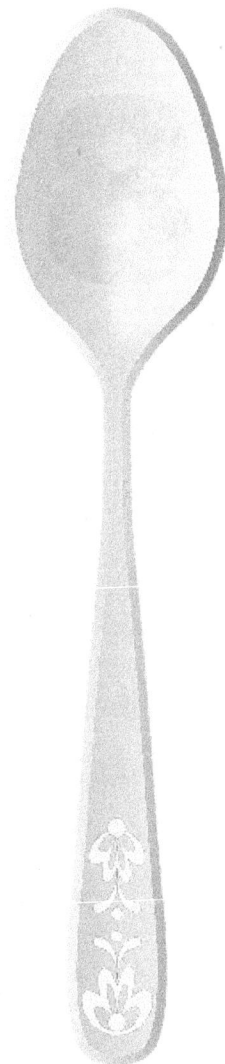

"The thirst mechanism in the brain is very effective at giving us a heads-up that it's time to hydrate."

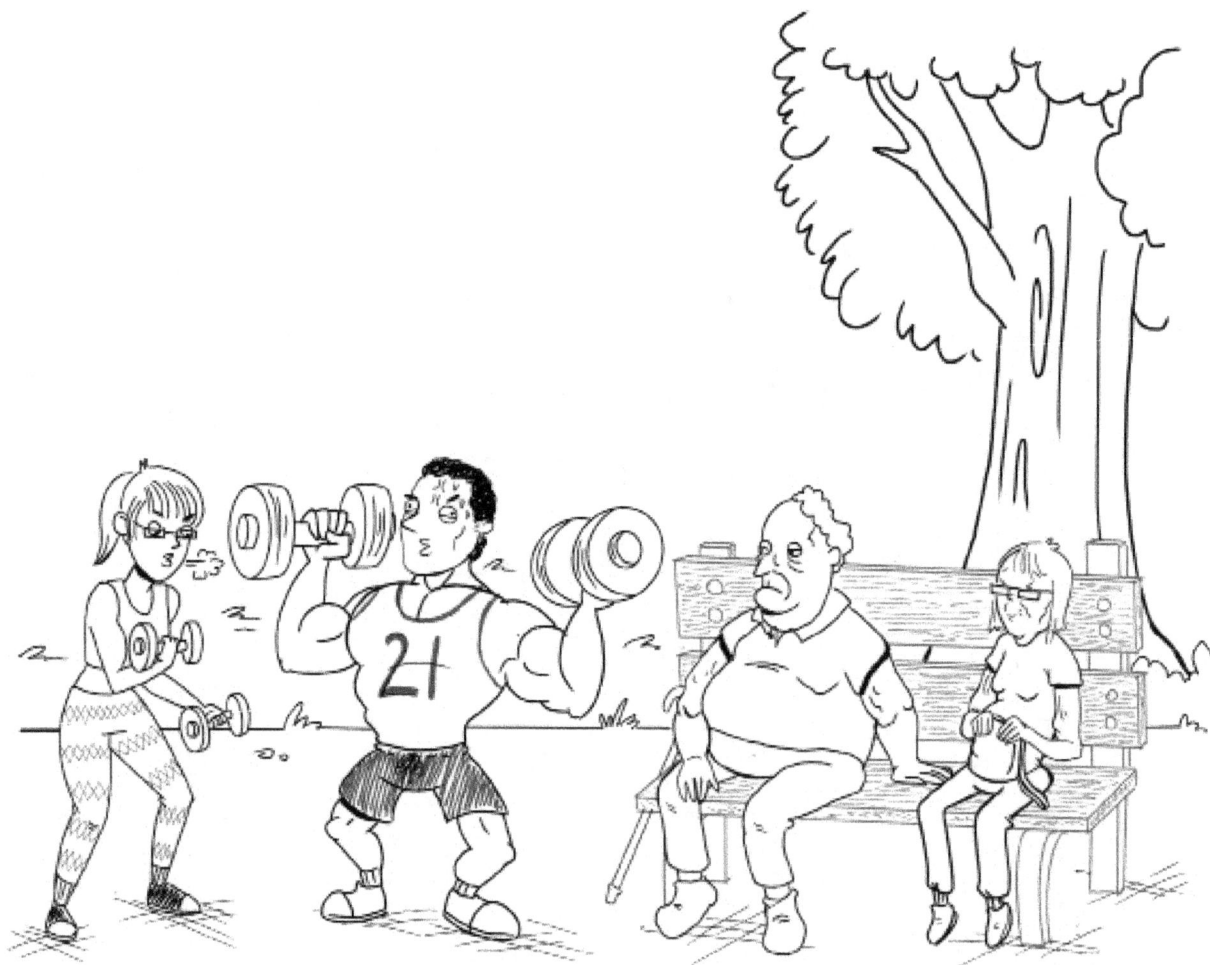

"Pump Up Now, So You Don't Plump Up Later."

MYTH Weight Gain is Inevitable as We Age

TRUTH A Healthy Diet and Regular Exercise Can Combat Weight Gain

9

YES, WE DO TEND TO PUT on weight as we age, but it's not inevitable. If you're in your forties or fifties and starting to put on weight, you need to make some simple lifestyle changes to reverse the situation. Don't use your age as an excuse!

One of the main reasons we gain weight in our golden years is that, from a distressingly early time of life, we begin losing muscle mass. This, in turn, causes our body's resting metabolic rate to decrease dramatically, which reduces the amount of calories (aka energy) we burn when we are standing, sitting or resting. This is why regular exercise as we age, in particular resistance training to build muscle mass, is so important.

Changes in our hormones mid-life also contribute to weight gain. For women, estrogen levels decrease dramatically. The body responds by retaining fat so that it can draw estrogen from fat cells. The result can be more belly fat. For men, the drop in testosterone levels can have the same effect. Eating more good fats such as polyunsaturated fats (essential fatty acids) and monounsaturated fats can help restore hormonal balance and stimulate the body's metabolism. Tuna, salmon and mackerel are oily fish that provide essential fatty acids. Seeds, nuts and olive oil are also good sources. Eating enough lean, quality proteins supports muscle regeneration.

Insulin resistance is another reason people put on belly fat in middle age. Insulin is a hormone that regulates the body's metabolism. Bad eating habits–such as a diet filled with refined carbohydrates–and carrying excess weight for too long can cause the body's insulin to become less effective (insulin resistance). This leaves excess glucose in the body, which is then stored as fat. You can keep your blood sugar levels in balance by adopting a healthier diet that is rich in legumes, vegetables, whole grains and other complex carbohydrates that contain fiber.

The key to maintaining a healthy body weight as you age is simple: continue to eat right and exercise regularly. Experts recommend 30 minutes of brisk walking four to five times a week and twice-weekly strength training to combat declining metabolic rates.

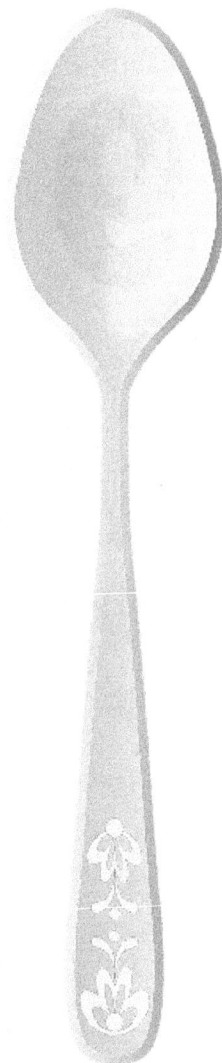

"If you're in your 40s or 50s and starting to put on weight, you need to make some simple lifestyle changes to reverse the situation."

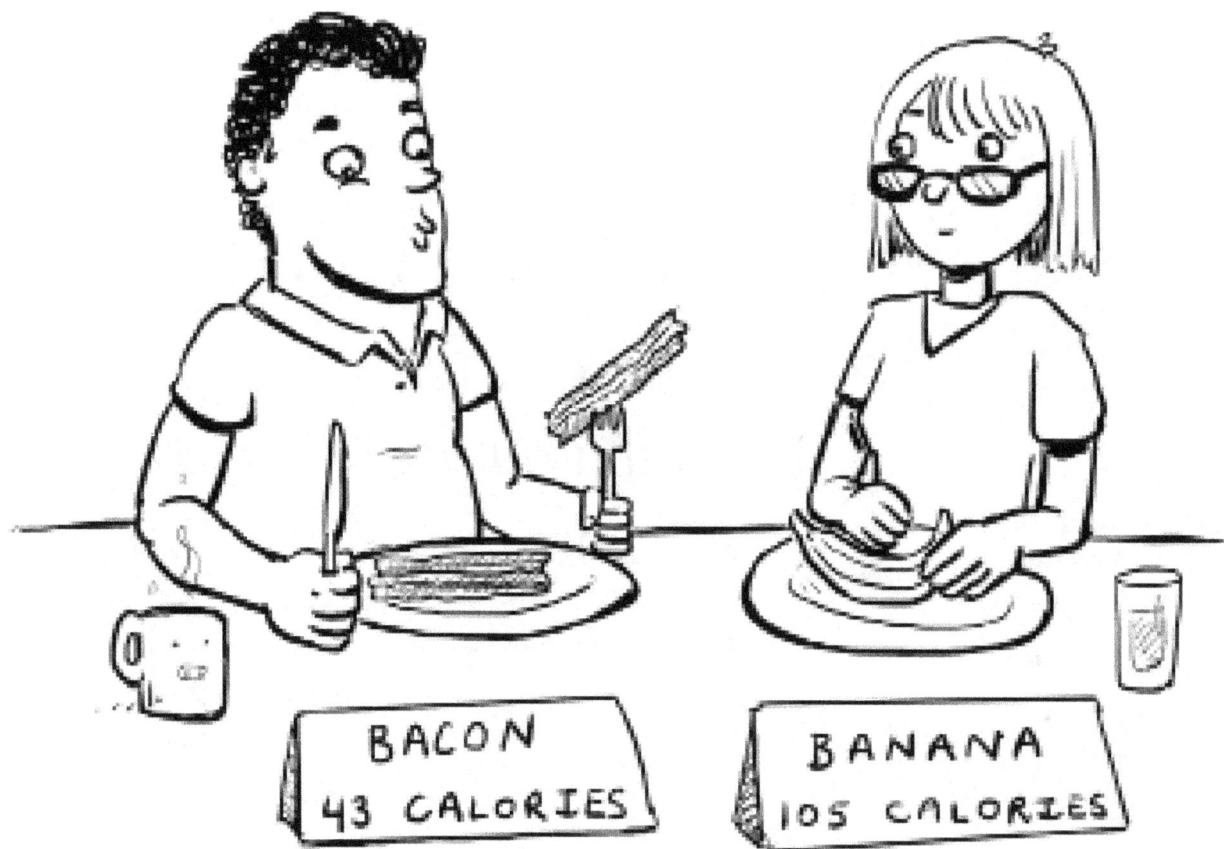

"When Calorie Counting Does Not Add Up."

MYTH All Calories Are Created Equal

TRUTH We Need a Mix of Foodstuffs for Optimal Health

AS A PRACTICING PHYSICIAN, I've heard it all when it comes to diet fads: the Vinegar Diet, the Nordic Diet, the Potato Chip Diet, the Keto Diet, the Ice Diet, the Paleo Diet, and the Baby Food Diet. There is even a Twinkie Diet, an Ice-Cream Cleanse, and a Cotton Ball Diet. In this last one, you eat cotton balls before meals to fill you up! I am not making this up.

People want to believe that if you eat one type of food, you can lose weight and live a healthy life. The truth is, man (and woman) cannot live on bread alone OR one type of calorie alone. Why? Because all calories are not created equal and we need a mix of calories for optimal health and wellbeing. No single food (or type of food) can provide all the nutrients you require as a human.

The word "calorie" denotes the amount of chemical energy stored in the food we eat. This energy is released through a range of biochemical processes, which we call our metabolism. There are three main types of macronutrient calories: proteins, carbohydrates and fats. Each is metabolized differently by the body and each plays a different role in human health. Your body needs some of each type of calorie—although nutritionists and researchers debate the optimal proportion and number of daily calories.

The human body can't stay healthy without a balance of calories from each of the macronutrient groups. Our bodies need us to ingest a variety of protein, carbohydrate and fat calories to support numerous functions in our circulatory, muscular, nervous, reproductive, skeletal and respiratory systems, among others. We metabolize fats differently from carbs and proteins because our body needs the range of energy and nutrients each provides. Sometimes, the specific combination of calorie types can be important. After an intense workout, for example, our bodies need more fluids, electrolytes and protein to replenish nutrients expended. Even geography and seasonal changes can influence the types of calories that should be consumed for optimal wellbeing. For example, if you live in a very cold climate, like Alaska, you might need more calories from foods like smoked salmon, which is rich in omega 3 fatty acids and supports skin integrity. Mushrooms, with their antiviral and antibacterial properties, might also be important in such a harsh climate as well as cheese for extra protein and Vitamin D, which can be lacking in winter months.

We metabolize food calories differently because that's what our body needs—variety and balance. Food calories can vary tremendously in their nutritional value, so listen to your body and ignore claims that the Twinkie Diet could change your life for the better. It can't!

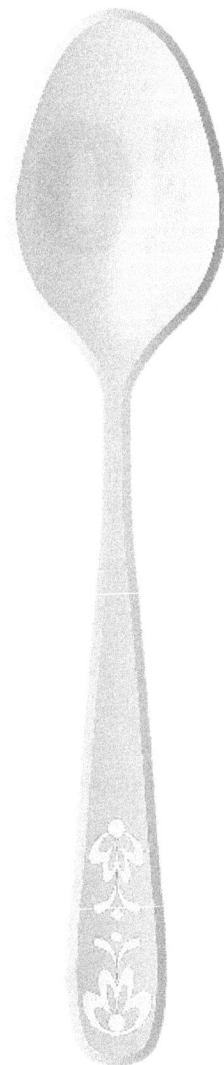

"No single food (or type of food) can provide all the nutrients you require."

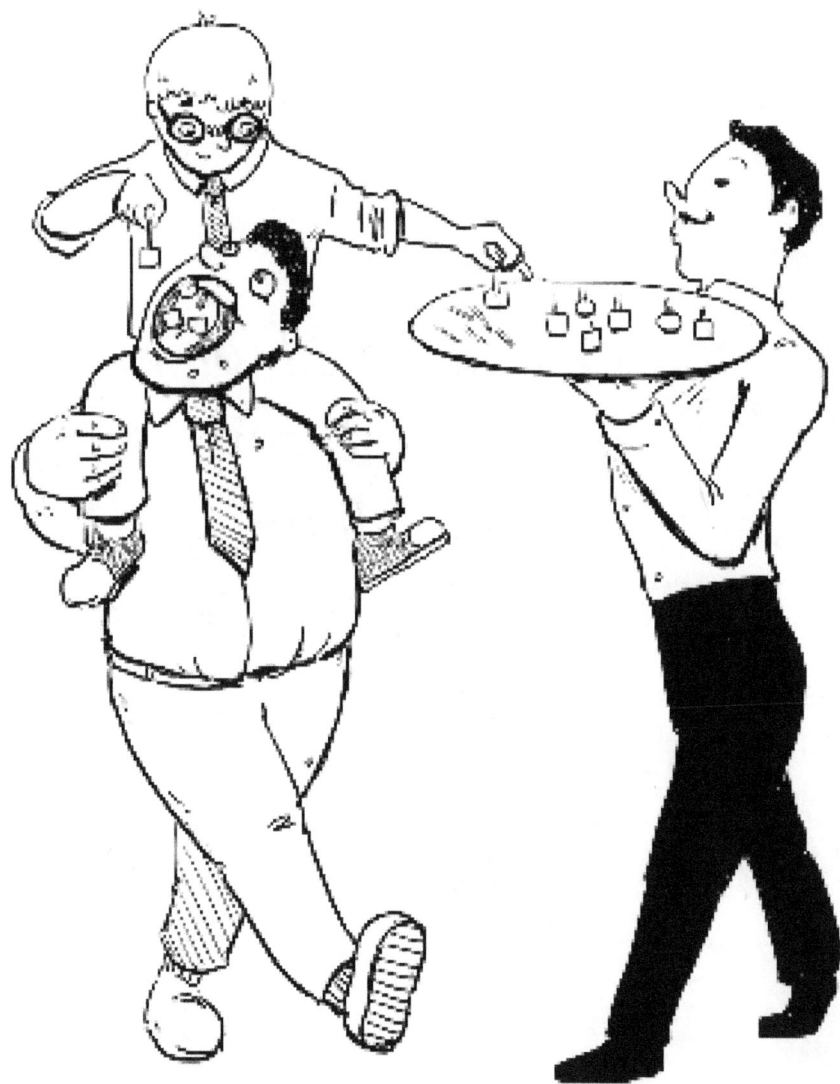

"Fill 'Er Up with Mini Cheese Bites, Please!"

MYTH 11

MYTH Eating Small Meals Throughout the Day Increases Metabolism

TRUTH Metabolism Is Impacted by the Size of Meals, Not the Number of Meals

NO ONE KNOWS HOW THIS myth started, but it's simply not true. Numerous scientific studies have shown that eating two to three meals per day has *the exact same effect on total calories burned* as eating five, six or more smaller meals. Frequent meals might help some people slake their hunger during the day, but it doesn't burn more calories. Some studies even show that eating too often can be counterproductive in terms of weight gain.

Our bodies do expend energy while digesting food. It's called the thermic effect of food (TEF). On average, the total TEF is around 10 percent of your total daily caloric intake. In other words, you burn about 10 percent of your calories *as* you eat. But studies show that eating six 500-calorie meals will cause the same thermic effect as eating three 1,000-calorie meals. Applying the average thermic effect of 10 percent, you'll burn 300 calories in both cases. When the number of calories consumed is the same, there is no difference in the metabolic rate, no matter how you slice it.

What can you do to boost your metabolism? Here are three ideas, all backed by science:

Add High Intensity Interval Training (HIIT) to your workout routine. HIIT has been shown to burn more fat and increase metabolic rate, even after finishing a workout. One study of overweight young men found that 12 weeks of high-intensity exercise had reduced their fat mass by more than 4 pounds and belly fat by 17 percent.

Stand more; sit less. One study showed that 185 minutes of standing as compared to sitting burned an extra 174 calories daily.

Get a good night's sleep. Lack of sleep has been cited as a major risk factor for obesity. It has also been linked to increased blood sugar levels and insulin resistance. As you might remember from an earlier myth, this can cause your body to store fat. Finally, lack of sleep has been shown to boost the hunger hormone ghrelin and decrease the fullness hormone leptin. This might explain why sleep-deprived people often feel hungry and struggle to lose weight.

Performance athletes and those who want to add muscle mass must consume more protein and sometimes more of certain carbohydrates in order to achieve their goals. Also, creatin, glutamine and other branch-chain amino acids are needed to achieve these goals—sometimes five or six times a day. However, the average person does not need to gain significant muscle mass in order to achieve optimal health. Small increases in muscle mass can improve a person's Resting Metabolic Rate (RMR), which is the number of calories your body burns while sitting, or at rest. Your RMR is influenced by your body's ratio of fat to muscle. This is where regular exercise comes into play in boosting your metabolism. Again, it all comes back to balance. Eat a balanced diet with a focus on nutrient-rich (not empty) calories, consume the right number of calories for your individual body type, get enough sleep and move regularly. This is how to achieve optimal health.

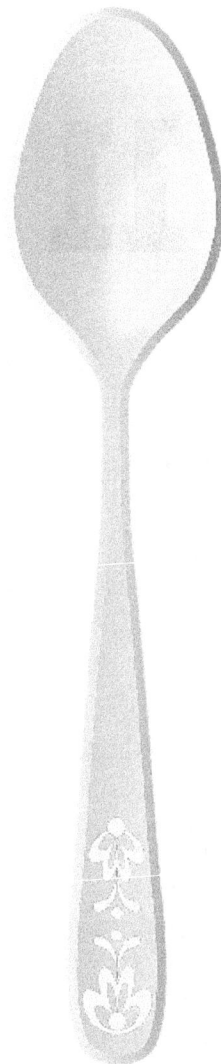

"Frequent meals might help some people slake their hunger during the day, but it doesn't burn more calories."

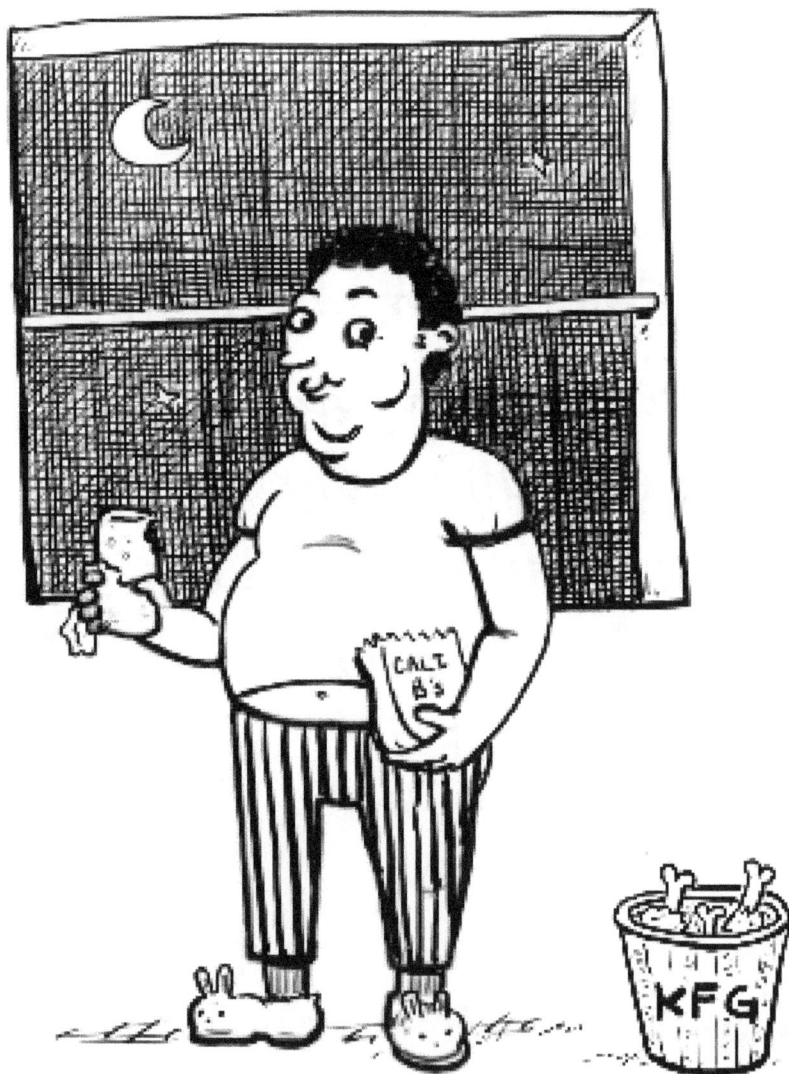

"Legend Has It That Every Full Moon, He Turns Into a Couch Potato."

MYTH Eating at Night Will Make You Fat

TRUTH Your Gut Is Not a Clock Watcher

It's not when you eat, it's *how much* you eat. "There is no magic hour in which your body decides that incoming calories must be stored as fat," says Jill Weisenberger, M.S., R.D., C.D.E., in an article for *Active*. If you routinely overindulge after dinner, it's the overindulging that's sabotaging your weight-control efforts, not the hour on the clock."

People assume that when you go to sleep your metabolism slows down and any leftover food in your stomach turns to fat. That's not how it works. During normal sleep, your metabolic rate does slow down by about 15 percent. But that doesn't mean your body decides to store calories as fat. Weight gain or loss is a pretty simple math equation: calories needed (based on age, activity level, and other factors) – calories consumed = weight gained or lost. Now, the ability to stick to that equation in order to lose weight can be sabotaged by your food choices and other factors, but that's a different story. If you're consuming highly processed foods with high levels of sugar, chances are you'll continue to crave nutrients that you're not providing to your body through those low-nutrition food choices. But if you make healthy food choices and follow the math, you will lose weight.

If you've been working out and consuming the right number of calories to achieve your weight goals, you'll be just fine. If you're sitting all day and overeating, you'll gain weight, no matter what time you eat that piece of chocolate cake.

"Sam Sells Expensive Sea Salts by the Seashore."

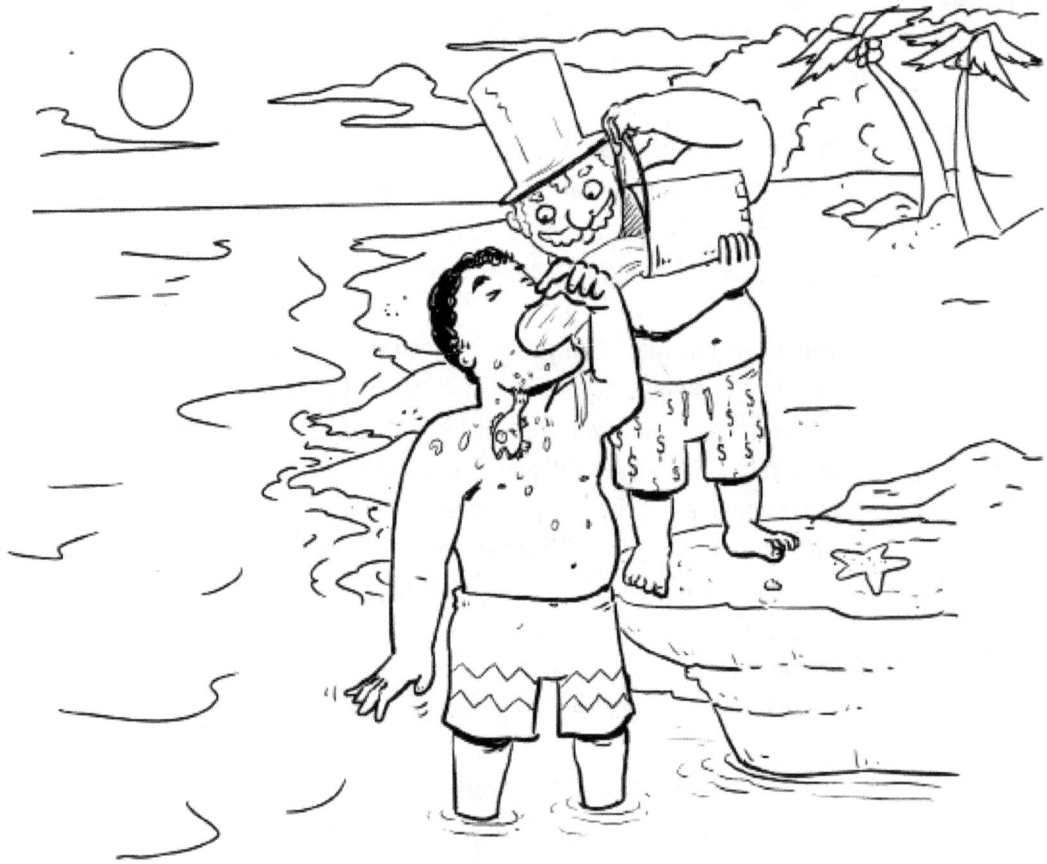

13

MYTH Sea Salt Is Better for You Than Table Salt

TRUTH Sea Salt Has Been Well Marketed

THE MAXIMUM RECOMMENDED DAILY INTAKE OF sodium is 2,300 milligrams. Guess what? One tablespoon of regular table salt contains roughly 2,300 milligrams of sodium, and one tablespoon of sea salt contains roughly 2,300 milligrams of sodium. No difference, except for the price. Sea salt and other gourmet salts cost exponentially more than standard table salt. But the only real differences between them are taste, texture and processing.

Because sea salt is minimally processed, it does retain a slightly higher level of certain minerals like magnesium and iron, but the vast majority of people get all the minerals they need from the foods they eat. Besides, you'd have to eat a couple of cups of sea salt each day to meet your minimum daily requirement of iron. You don't need to be a nutritionist to understand that this wouldn't be a healthy choice.

The real issue for most Americans is not which type of salt they use, but having too much sodium. Table salt is about 40 percent sodium and 60 percent chloride, a mineral. But salt isn't the big culprit in America's sodium overdose. Sodium is a cheap and very popular food additive. It is included in many food preservatives and flavor enhancers. Because of its widespread use, most Americans consume way too much of it.

Excess sodium increases blood pressure because it holds excess fluid in the body, and that creates an added burden on the heart. Too much sodium increases the risk of stroke, heart failure, osteoporosis, stomach cancer and kidney disease.

When you're sprinkling sea salt instead of table salt, you might be tempted to think you're putting something healthier on your corn on the cob or potato. Truth is, you're not.

According to Katherine Zeratsky, R.D., L.D., of the Mayo Clinic, "Sea salt and table salt have the same basic nutritional value, despite the fact that sea salt is often promoted as being healthier. Sea salt and table salt contain comparable amounts of sodium by weight." Her advice and mine? Whichever type of salt you use to flavor your food, sprinkle in moderation.

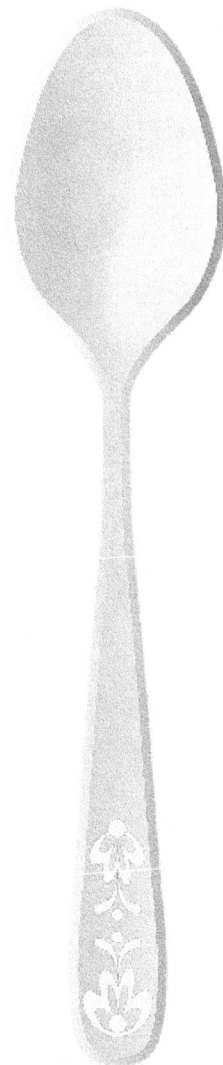

"The real issue
for most Americans is
not which type
of salt they use, but
having too
much sodium."

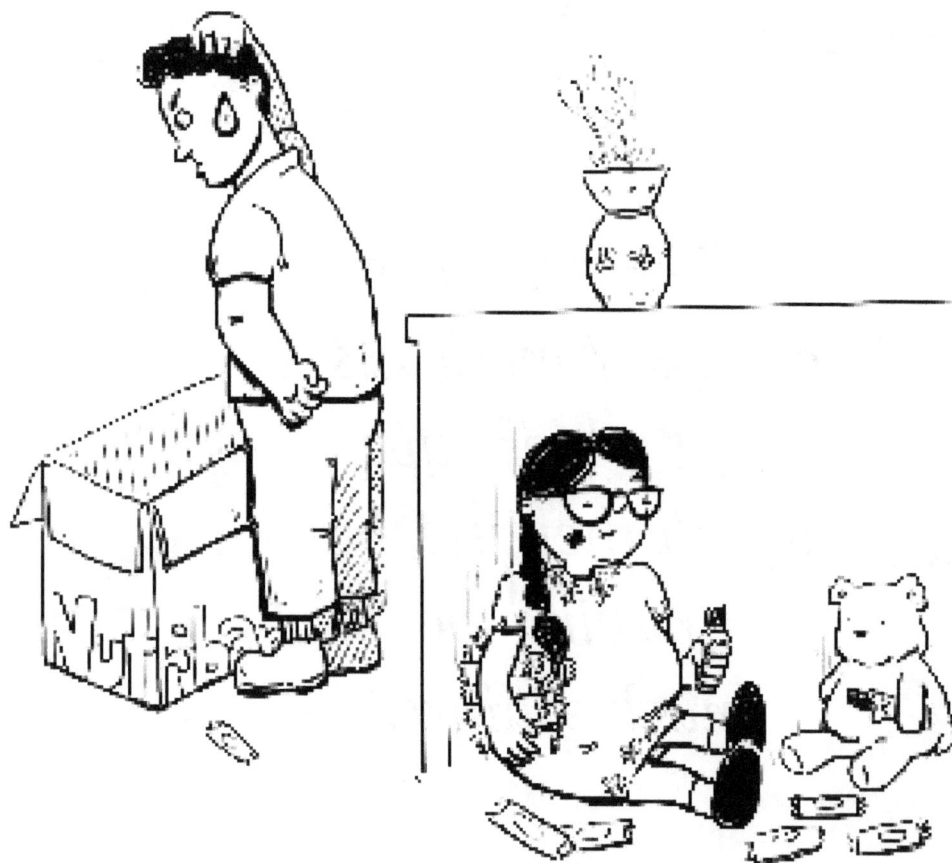

"Where Did All the Energy Bars Go?"

MYTH Energy Bars Are Nutritious

TRUTH Most Energy Bars Are Like Candy Bars

14

The advertising budgets that drive the $5.1 billion energy bar market are huge. Truth is, most energy bars are just candy bars dressed up to look healthy with fancy wrappers. Sure, there are a few nutritional bar brands that are pretty well balanced and contain few or no processed additives–but that's the exception, not the rule.

"In a world where we really call it as it is," says David Zinczenko, author of the bestselling *Eat This, Not That! Series* and *Men's Fitness* editorial director, "nutrition bars would be known by another name: calorie bars. Most of them are so polluted with additives that their ingredients list looks like Charlie Sheen's blood test results."

So how do you know which bars to eat when you are hungry and on the go? Assume the worst and take a moment to check out the number of calories in the bar and see if it contains unhealthy ingredients like hydrogenated or partially hydrogenated oils or corn syrup. I think you'll be shocked by what you find on the nutrition panel for many of these bars.

Helen Mullen, a certified dietitian nutritionist and a clinical dietitian with New York-Presbyterian, provided this guidance in an article from *Health Matters*: "The fewer ingredients on the label, the better. The more additives you see–particularly excess sugar alcohols (sorbitol, xylitol), which can cause gastric distress–the less likely the bar is to deserve the 'healthy' moniker. Palm oils, soy protein isolate and so-called natural flavors are also red flags. Instead, reach for a bar with fewer ingredients and make sure you recognize them and can pronounce them."

Okay, I get it. In my hectic day, I like to grab something quick with a decent amount of protein to tide me over. Sometimes, I do grab an energy bar for lunch. Mostly, though, I choose a healthier alternative. Here are some of my favorite healthy snack options: a handful of mixed nuts, a bag of dried fruit and nut mix, a snack-size can of tuna, or a small container of low-fat cottage cheese.

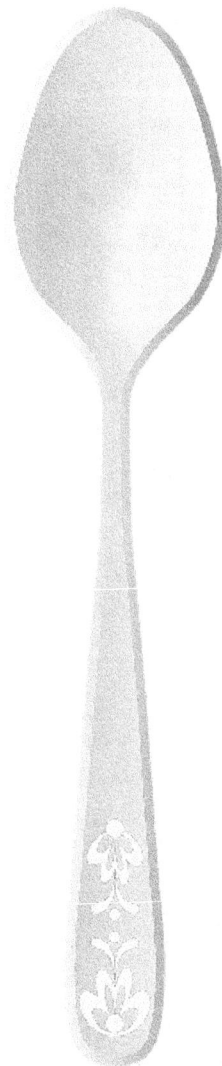

"Most energy bars are just candy bars dressed up to look healthy with fancy wrappers."

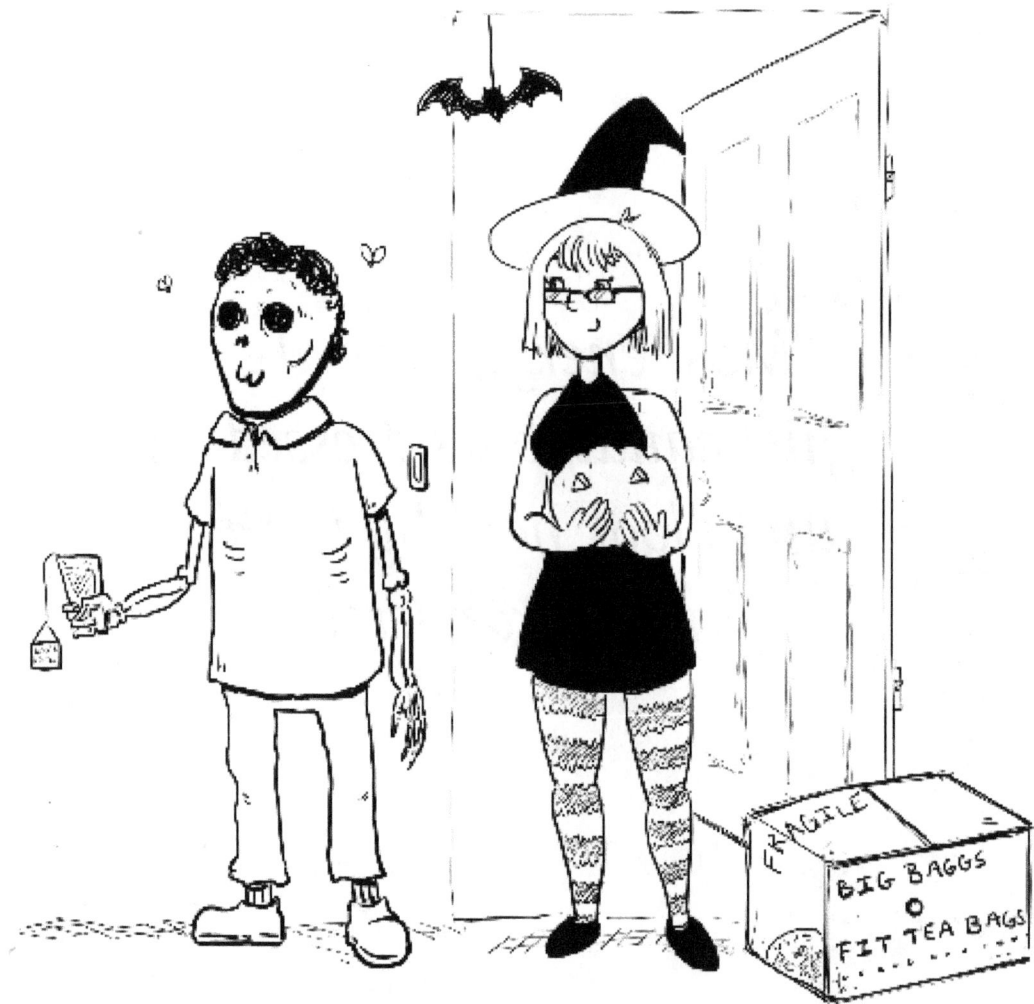

"I Guess There Will Be No Treats for You This Halloween, Honey!"

15

MYTH Starvation Diets Are a Good Way To Lose Weight

TRUTH Prolonged Starvation Diets Are Dangerous

STARVATION DIETS HAVE BEEN AROUND for a long time and continue to be popular with people who want to lose weight fast. During a starvation diet, food intake and calories are highly restricted to 300 to 700 calories a day. Research indicates that people who eat 50 percent of their energy needs for three weeks do decrease their body weight overall. But this quick weight loss often comes with some dangerous side effects.

According to an article in *InBody* that spotlighted a number of scientific studies, "If the state of starvation is maintained chronically, lean muscle mass and organ size are decreased by 20 percent....Weight loss via starvation causes individuals to lose significant amounts of lean muscle mass to and lean body mass, which encompasses water, bones, organs, etc. Reducing the mass of your bones is problematic, as that decreases bone density and can make you more prone to injury."

As a practicing physician, one of my worries is that if people do not get enough protein for their bodies to meet their energy needs during a period of fasting, they can disturb their metabolism and their health. Many of my patients claim that they fast to "detox" their bodies. But, as humans, we already have wonderful systems and organs to help us "detox" on a regular basis. These organs include our kidneys, liver, colon, and skin. If you keep these organs healthy, they'll continue detoxifying your body whether you are fasting or not.

Though I am not an advocate of long-term fasting, some of my patients appear to have benefited from short-term fasts that last a day or two. They lose a few pounds as a result of their short fast and this gives them a degree of confidence that they can continue to lose weight. They have better mental clarity that may help them initiate and commit to a more sustained weight-loss program. I tell them that they can also benefit from a two-day meditation retreat to gain mental clarity and focus for their weight-loss goal. Other patients, however, have negative side effects, especially from longer fasts. Several patients have told me they lost a few pounds through intermittent fasting, only to rebound and gain most of the pounds back when they reverted to a regular eating schedule. Another patient reported sleep issues during her fast. Studies do indicate that prolonged fasting can decrease the length and quality of sleep.

But short-term fasting is different than long-term fasting, which is a form of starvation. Not only is starving yourself dangerous, in a great twist of irony, it can often lead to *weight gain* over time. How? By changing your metabolism. When you try to return to a normal caloric intake, your body can't handle it. Starvation trains your body to have lower metabolism and when you start eating again, you end up gaining weight, even on a normal diet. During the starvation diet, you've trained your body to store fat, and it's not going to forget that lesson. Now, whenever your body gets its hands on a few extra calories, it will store those calories as fat.

Starvation mode is the body's mechanism for dealing with emergencies (like famine). It's not meant to be a long-term state. Our bodies need a certain amount of vitamins, minerals, and protein every day. According to Mikel Byrant, a nutritionist at the Mayo Clinic, fasting for an extended period of time is not recommended, especially for those under 18 years of age, physically active adults, pregnant women or those with medical conditions.

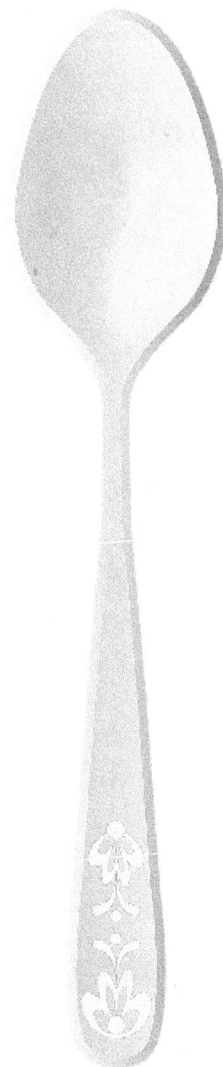

"Weight loss via starvation causes individuals to lose significant amounts of lean muscle mass."

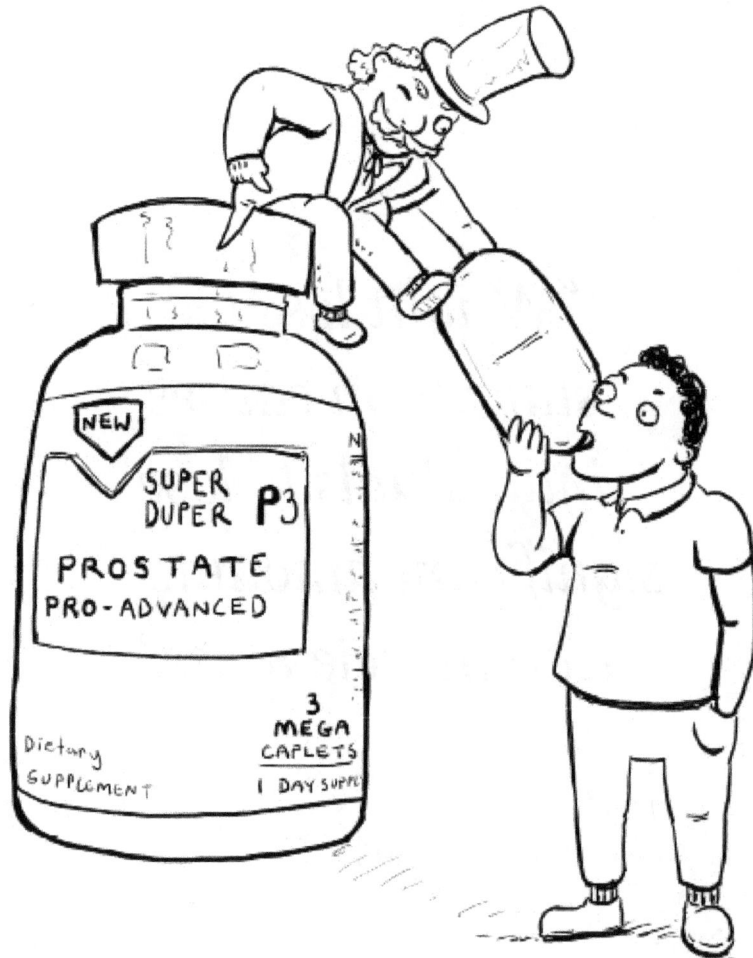

"Just Swallow Three a Day."

16

MYTH Prostate Supplements Can Prevent Cancer

TRUTH No Over-the-counter or Prescription Drug Prevents Prostate Cancer

IN RECENT YEARS, DOZENS IF NOT hundreds of homeopathic male supplements have hit the market. Many of these supplements claim to contain proprietary blends of nature-derived ingredients and minerals that can reduce trips to the bathroom, reduce middle-of-the-night wake-ups, and support prostate function. There is some valid clinical evidence that these claims are true—at least to some extent, in some patients, and for a certain period of time. But there is absolutely no clinically valid evidence that any of them prevent prostate cancer. The Prostate Cancer Foundation confirms: "Although significant progress has been made and genetic and environmental risk factors for prostate cancer have been identified, the evidence is not strong enough for conclusive recommendations on prostate cancer prevention."

Despite an absence of evidence that these supplements prevent cancer, the market continues to grow for prostate health products. Is there any harm in this, even if people are ultimately just throwing their money away? In general, no; in reality, perhaps. If people believe that these supplements are all they need to keep their bodies healthy, they might overlook other things they should be doing to prevent cancer. Here are the American Cancer Society's general recommendations:

- Eat a diet rich in fiber
- Consume at least two-and-a-half cups of vegetables and fruits each day
- Choose whole grains products over those made with refined grains
- Limit alcohol to one drink a day for women and two drinks a day for men
- Avoid processed meats and limit the amount of red meat that you eat

The lucrative supplement market targets many types of cancer fear with their prevention claims. But, as with the Prostate Cancer supplements, the claims don't hold up under scrutiny. The Rogel Cancer Center at the University of Michigan looked at 10 supplements, including fish oil, flaxseed and ginger supplements. None of their studies resulted in any conclusive evidence that these supplements could prevent cancer. The Rogel Cancer Center reiterated the fact that following the healthy-diet guidelines recommended by the American Cancer Society are the best way to prevent cancer.

In a product review of 16 prostate supplements, ConsumerLabs stated that none of the supplement products it reviewed appeared to prevent prostate cancer, and "Certain products also appear to violate FDA rules for what should (and should not) be on labels."

These are the myths that do not sit well with me or many of my medical colleagues. Claims of cancer prevention should not be made lightly and certainly not without extensive scientific research to support such claims. In my experience, such claims cause patients to develop a false sense of security. They skip their annual physicals and forgo proven screening test like the digital prostate exam or PSA test (which tests for levels of prostate specific antigens) because they feel "protected" by unproven supplements that promise more than they can deliver. It's unsettling as a doctor to watch these scenarios unfold because early detection is key to survival in many types of cancer.

The reality is that no other over-the-counter or prescription drug can prevent prostate cancer, so PLEASE get screened regularly and talk to your doctor if your prostate health changes. The National Cancer Institute lists the following signs and symptoms that may be caused by prostate cancer. Check with your doctor if you have any of the following:

- Weak or interrupted ("stop-and-go") flow of urine.
- Sudden urge to urinate.
- Frequent urination (especially at night).
- Trouble starting the flow of urine.
- Trouble emptying the bladder completely.
- Pain or burning while urinating.
- Blood in the urine or semen.

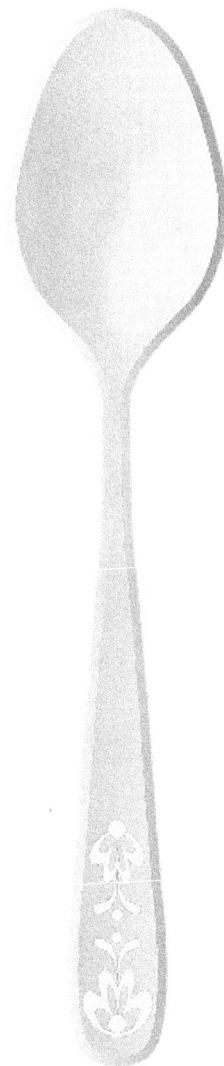

- A pain in the back, hips, or pelvis that doesn't go away.
- Shortness of breath, feeling very tired, fast heartbeat, dizziness, or pale skin caused by anemia

Here is a bit of common sense: establish a strong relationship with your primary care doctor and see him or her regularly—not just when you are sick. Don't skip your annual physical exam and health screenings. Your primary care doctor is the best person to guide you. He or she has seen, diagnosed, and treated cancers of all sorts. Every day, your doctor works closely with cancer-specialists to care for patients and administer preventive tests. One final thought: Have a conversation about the important topic of cancer prevention and preventive supplements with your doctor rather than blindly believing a supplement company's claims. It could be a life-saving exchange.

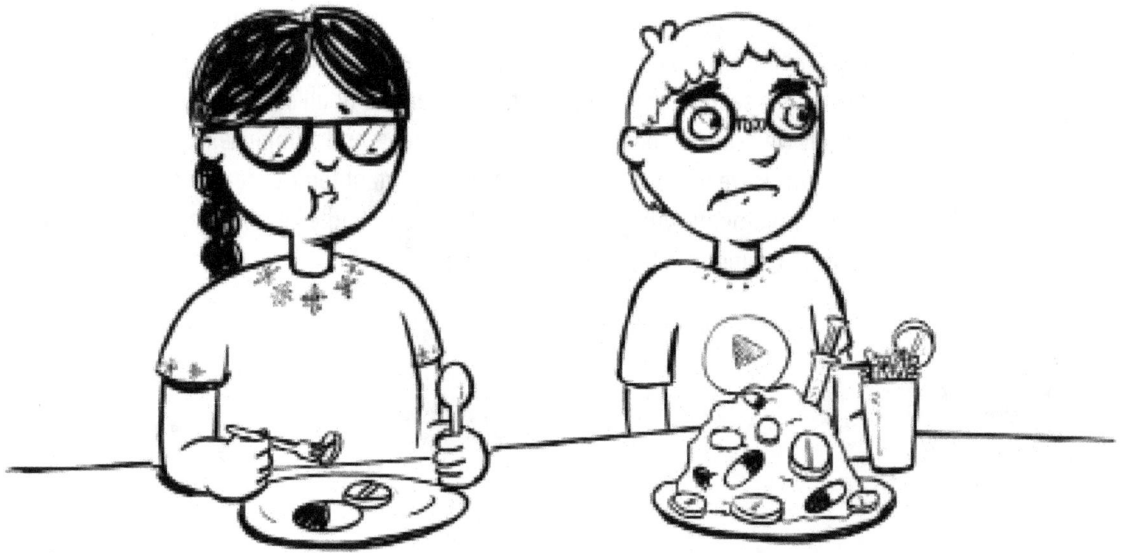

"Welcome to Mount Pillmore!"

17

MYTH With Nutraceuticals, More Is Better

TRUTH Consuming Too Many Nutraceuticals Can Harm You

IF SOME NUTRACEUTICALS ARE GOOD, more must be better, right? That's what many Americans believe as they continue to gobble up more and more of these supplements. The term "nutraceutical" was coined in 1989 by Stephen De Felice, founder and chairman of the Foundation for Innovation in Medicine. He defined a nutraceutical as a "food, or parts of a food, that provide medical or health benefits, including the prevention and treatment of disease." In short, nutraceutical is mostly a fancy word for vitamin, herbal or mineral supplements.

You can't take too many vitamins, right? If you ingest more than your body actually needs, they'll just "pass through." Vitamin, herbal, and mineral supplements aren't drugs, so they can't harm you. That's what all too many Americans believe. But, sorry, those statements are just not accurate.

Hypervitaminosis is one example of too much of a good thing. Hypervitaminosis A, for example, is a condition that occurs when a person has too much vitamin A in his or her body. This can happen if a person takes too many supplements or uses certain creams for acne over a prolonged period. Symptoms of Hypervitaminosis A include vision problems, changes to the skin, and bone pain. Chronic cases of Hypervitaminosis A may result in liver damage, which is not always reversible.

Because nutraceuticals are self-prescribed, inappropriate use, overdose and interactions with other medicines are always a possibility. According to *The Pharmaceutical Journal*, consumers "are unaware of the difference between licensed and unlicensed products, and the differences between food legislation and medicine legislation. There are many inaccurate claims made for many supplements available, as well as much variation in the actual products, depending on storage, manufacturing process, or even batches of the same material. It is vital that these discrepancies be resolved, possibly with the creation of a third type of regulatory category for supplements."

Americans want a pill for everything. As a nation, we are obsessed with pills. Nutraceutical company reps come to my office and try to sell me pills that have all the nutrients of an orange. What would my patients miss if they skipped the orange and took the pill? They would miss the important fiber found in the orange, which can lower cholesterol in the blood and prevent colon cancer.

Nutraceuticals can play a role in human health. For example, if your iron levels are low, taking an iron supplement is probably wise. But make sure to let your doctor know what nutraceuticals you are taking, especially if you are also taking prescription medications or suffer from any long-term health conditions or illnesses. Otherwise, don't overindulge in nutraceuticals. There is simply no substitute for a well-balanced diet. It is the ideal source of vitamins and minerals and rarely over-delivers (or under-delivers) nutrients the way nutraceuticals can.

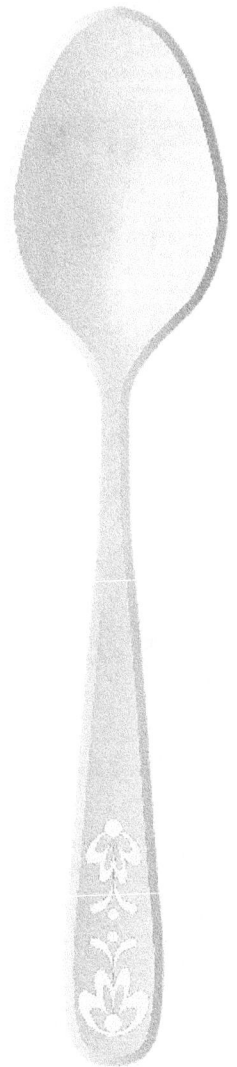

*"Hypervitaminosis
is one example
of too much of
a good thing."*

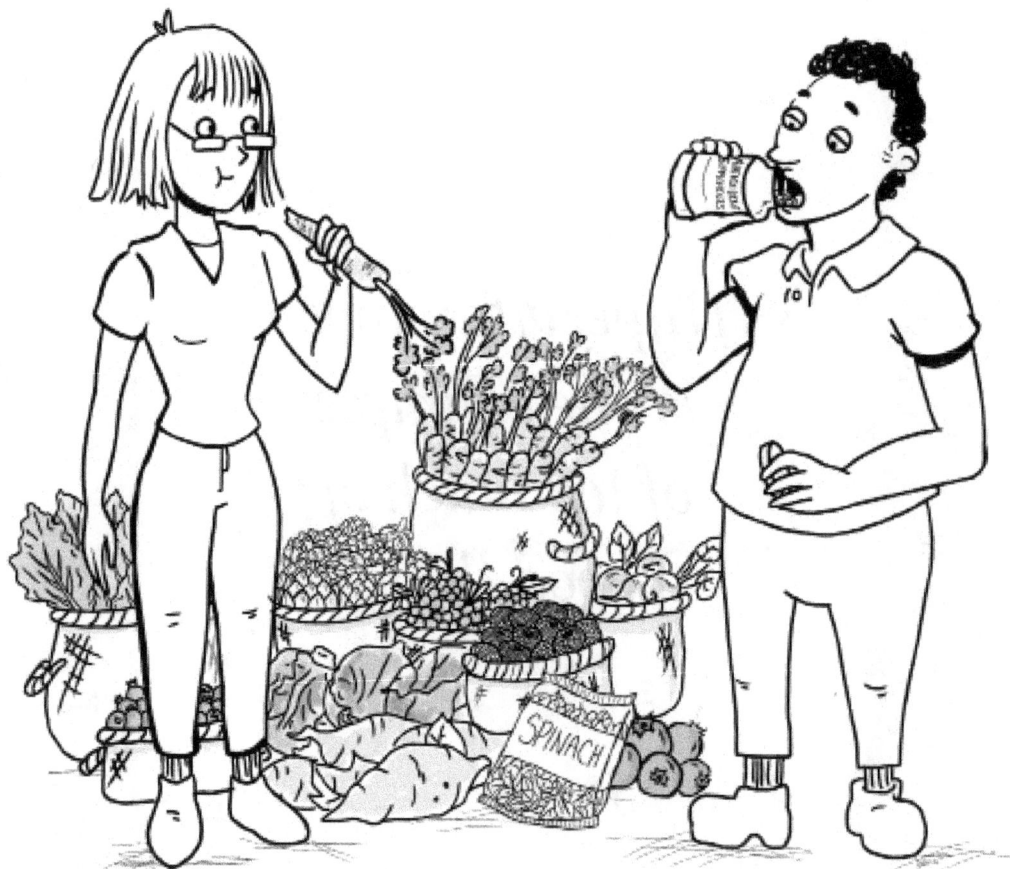

"Take That, Cancer Cells!"

MYTH Eating Foods High in Antioxidants Prevents Cancer

TRUTH Antioxidants Have Benefits But Cancer Prevention Has Not Been Proven

18

While there's plenty of scientific research to suggest that antioxidants are enormously useful in neutralizing free radicals (molecules in our bloodstream that are thought to be culprits in a host of diseases like Alzheimer's), there is no conclusive scientific evidence that supplementing the human diet with foods high in antioxidants has the power to prevent cancer. In fact, a growing number of studies indicate that antioxidants appear to make some cancers worse!

An article in *Scientific American* states the conundrum on antioxidants: "The conventional wisdom is that antioxidants should lower cancer risk by neutralizing cell-damaging, cancer-causing free radicals. But scientists now think that antioxidants, at high enough levels, also protect cancer cells from these same free radicals. 'There now exists a sizable quantity of data suggesting that antioxidants can help cancer cells much like they help normal cells,' says Zachary Schafer, a biologist at the University of Notre Dame."

If you want to prevent cancer, here are the top 7 tips suggested by the Mayo Clinic:

1. Don't use tobacco
2. Eat a healthy diet (no that's not a contradiction; a good diet has many health benefits)
3. Maintain a healthy weight and be physically active
4. Protect yourself from the sun
5. Get vaccinated
6. Avoid risky behaviors that can lead to infections
7. Get regular medical care

I agree with all of these recommendations and encourage you to have a heart-to-heart conversation with your doctor about what other lifestyle adjustments could help prevent cancer. All of our physiologies, lifestyle choices, and family histories are unique, so it's best to have this talk with your family doctor. He or she knows you and your system best.

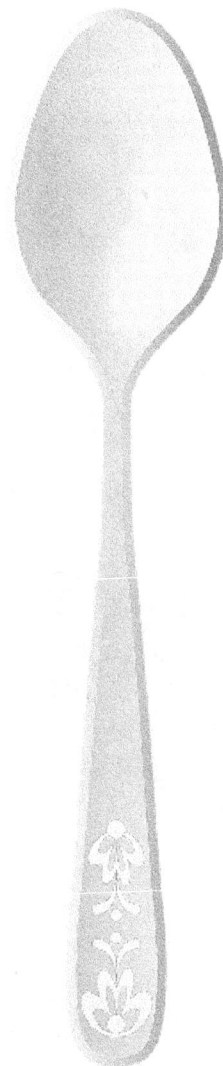

"Have a heart-toheart conversation with your doctor about what other lifestyle adjustments could help prevent cancer."

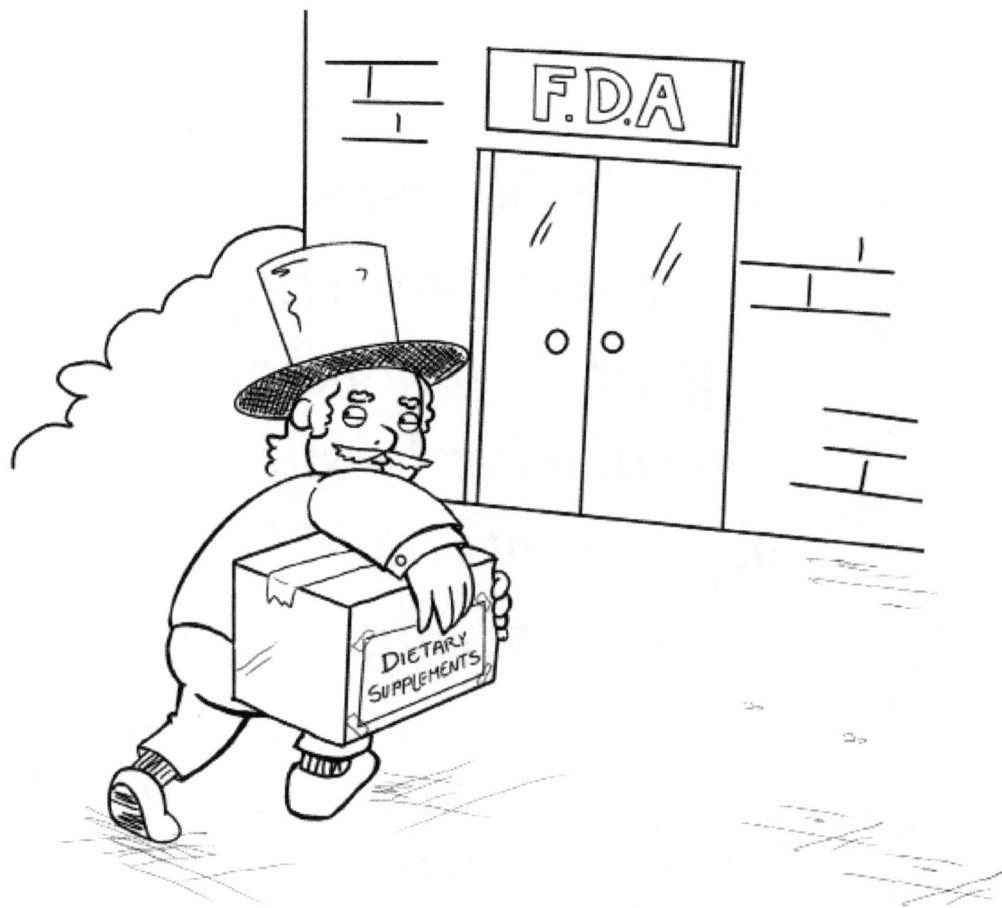

"I Ain't Afraid of No Ghosts or the FDA!"

MYTH Dietary Supplements Are Safe Because They Are FDA-Approved

TRUTH Dietary Supplements Are Not Regulated by the FDA

LET ME BE VERY CLEAR, the Food and Drug Administration (FDA) *does not* regulate over-the-counter dietary supplements and this is a big problem for consumers. It can be dangerous to assume that all dietary supplements are safe without FDA oversight. However, the FDA *does* provide a number of guidelines for manufacturers, particularly with respect to product labeling. But even when a product meets the FDA's guidelines, the labels must still carry this caveat about the product's efficacy and benefits: *"These statements have not been evaluated by the FDA."*

Three out of four Americans now consume supplements regularly. Understand, however, that if you are buying a dietary supplement that makes a claim like "prevents the free radicals that cause cancer," there is probably no scientific evidence to support that claim and the FDA has not vetted the claim to see if it is valid. There is a ridiculous amount of false advertising in the dietary supplements market.

In February 2019, FDA Commissioner Scott Gottlieb, M.D., released a statement about the agency's new efforts to strengthen regulation of dietary supplements by modernizing and reforming FDA's oversight. In the statement, Gottlieb recognized that the FDA "plays an important role in helping consumers make use of safe, high-quality dietary supplements while also protecting Americans from the potential dangers of products that don't meet the agency's standards for marketing. In the 25 years since Congress passed the Dietary Supplement Health and Education Act (DSHEA), the law that transformed the FDA's authority to regulate dietary supplements, the dietary supplement market has grown significantly. What was once a $4 billion industry comprised of about 4,000 unique products, is now an industry worth more than $40 billion, with more than 50,000–and possibly as many as 80,000 or more–different products available to consumers."

If you are taking dietary supplements on a regular basis, I strongly suggest you research the FDA's guidance on supplements. Among other things, the FDA suggests you consult with a health-care provider before using any dietary supplement. Additionally, the FDA advises: "Many supplements contain ingredients that have strong biological effects, and such products may not be safe in all people. If you have certain health conditions and take these products, you may be putting yourself at risk." The government organization also states:

- Dietary supplements are not intended to treat, diagnose, cure, or alleviate the effects of diseases.
- Using supplements improperly can be harmful.
- Some supplements can have unwanted effects before, during, or after surgery.

The dietary supplement market is like the Wild West. Luckily, it looks like the recent FDA sheriffs are working to reign things in and better regulate the supplement market. Let's hope so. As a consumer, you need to do your part as well. Make sure you look at consumer reports about the track record of supplement companies and ask a lot of questions before buying or ingesting any supplements. Finally, do not try to hide your use of supplements or herbs from your doctor. Vitamins, minerals, and herbal supplements can sometimes have serious interactions with your prescription medications.

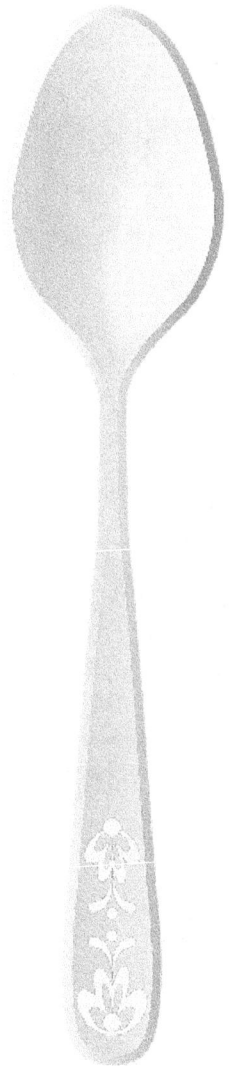

"The dietary supplement market is like the Wild West."

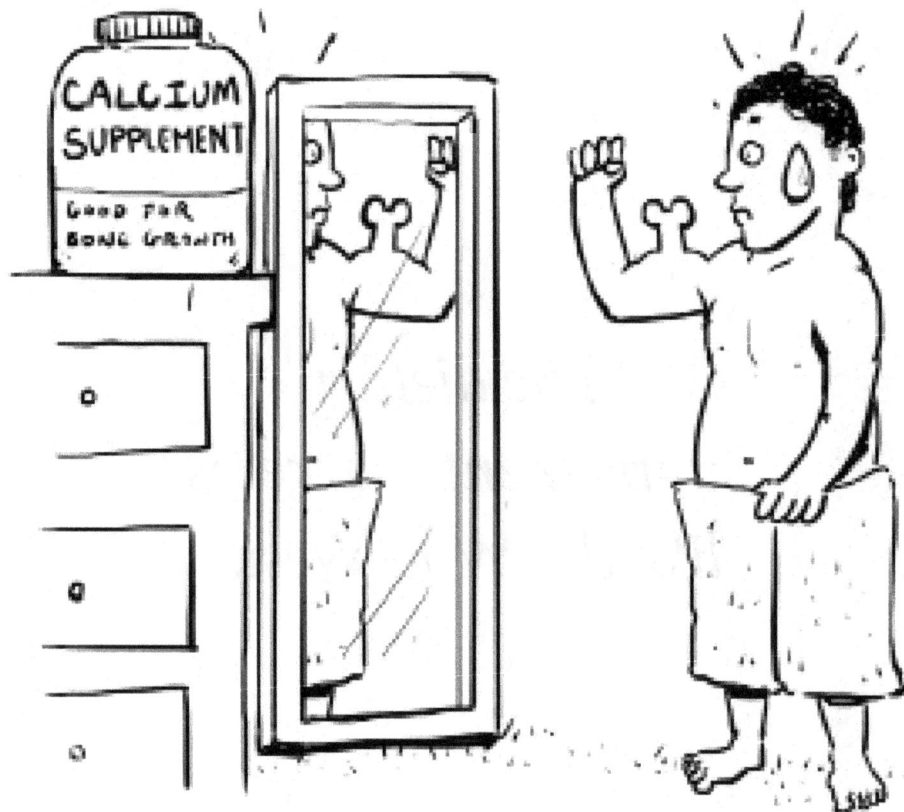

"Yikes! How Did This Happen?"

MYTH You Can't Take Too Much Calcium

TRUTH Too Much Calcium Can Harm You

20

YEP, IT'S TRUE, TOO MUCH calcium may harm your health. Calcium plays a critical role in our diet, helping us to build and maintain health bones. You'd think that calcium would be benign, even in very high doses. It's not. Too much calcium can actually be dangerous.

Dr. Melissa Young of the Cleveland Clinic says that "More and more studies are showing increased risks for heart attack and stroke among men and women taking calcium 1,000 to 1,200 milligrams (mg) per day, which was previously recommended." According to the same Cleveland Clinic article, "Researchers believe that without adequate Vitamin D to help absorb it, the extra calcium settles in the arteries, instead of the bones. There, it helps form plaques that threaten the heart and brain. Excess calcium can also cause muscle pain, mood disorders, abdominal pain and kidney stones."

Like me, Dr. Young recommends obtaining the majority of your calcium needs from foods. The body absorbs and utilizes calcium better from foods. Here's a list of highly absorbable sources of calcium:

- Leafy green vegetables like spinach and kale
- Legumes and beans
- Sardines and salmon
- Sesame seeds
- Fortified foods, like milk and orange juice

Maybe you're thinking, that's a long list of foods to remember if I want to get in all the important nutrients I need. Well, to keep it simple, follow the Mediterranean diet. It has most of these calcium-rich foods and is rated as one of the best weight loss and wellness diets on the planet. It is designed to meet all of your vitamin, mineral, protein and fiber needs.

I have been on a long academic journey since med school to keep current with the nutrition research literature. That's 20 years of watching nutritional trends as a practicing physician. In the end, my parents were right, you can stay healthy by eating a well-balanced diet filled with a variety of fresh, healthy foods. It's simpler than you think. Thanks, Mom and Dad!

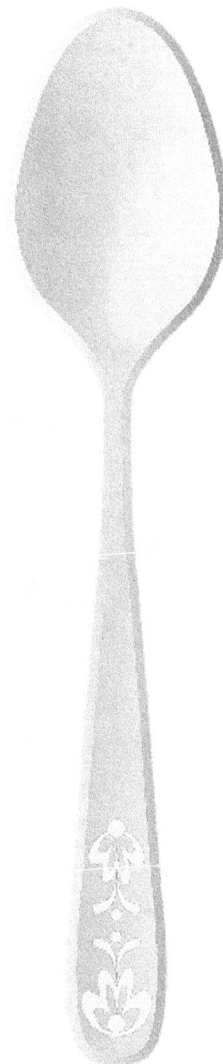

"Excess calcium can cause muscle pain, mood disorders, abdominal pain and kidney stones."

"Who Has Time to Dry Their Hair?!"

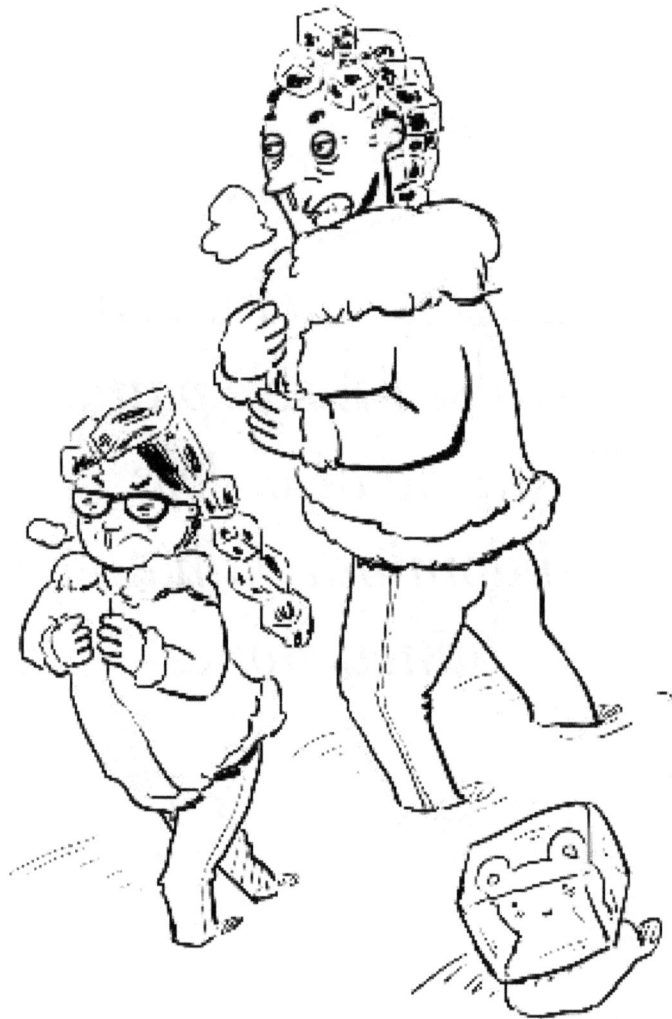

21

MYTH You'll Get Sick if You Go Out in the Cold With Wet Hair

TRUTH You'll Be Fine! Enjoy the Outdoors With Wet or Dry Hair

THERE'S NOT A BIT OF TRUTH to this old wives' tale that you'll get sick if you go out in the cold with wet hair! It's hard to know when this myth first took flight, but it was undoubtedly a very long time ago. Colds are caused by a virus being transmitted from person to person–period, end of story! Sorry, this one makes me a little crazy.

While it is true that the human body is generally under more stress in the wintertime than in other seasons, most people deal with winter just fine. It's also true that *ultra*-cold weather is a big stressor on the body, and hypothermia can definitely suppress your immune system enough to make you more vulnerable to colds. But unless you're washing your hair in the Arctic, the winter and wet hair combination isn't the danger your grandma told you it was.

The actual reason why we get sick in the winter is that we are indoors more often and thus share germs more often. Getting the flu shot and encouraging those close to you to get the flu shot will provide what's called a "blue zone of immunity" for your group. Also, controlling stress is important because it can bring down your immune system and make you more susceptible to winter bugs.

Many patients ask me how to stay well in the winter. Nobel Laureate Linus Pauling believed Vitamin C was the answer. From where I sit as a practicing physician who sees patients throughout the cold and flu season, Vitamin C is not the answer. Take it if you think it helps, but my advice to my patients is simple: get enough sleep, practice good hand hygiene, eat well, exercise, and be careful around those who are sick.

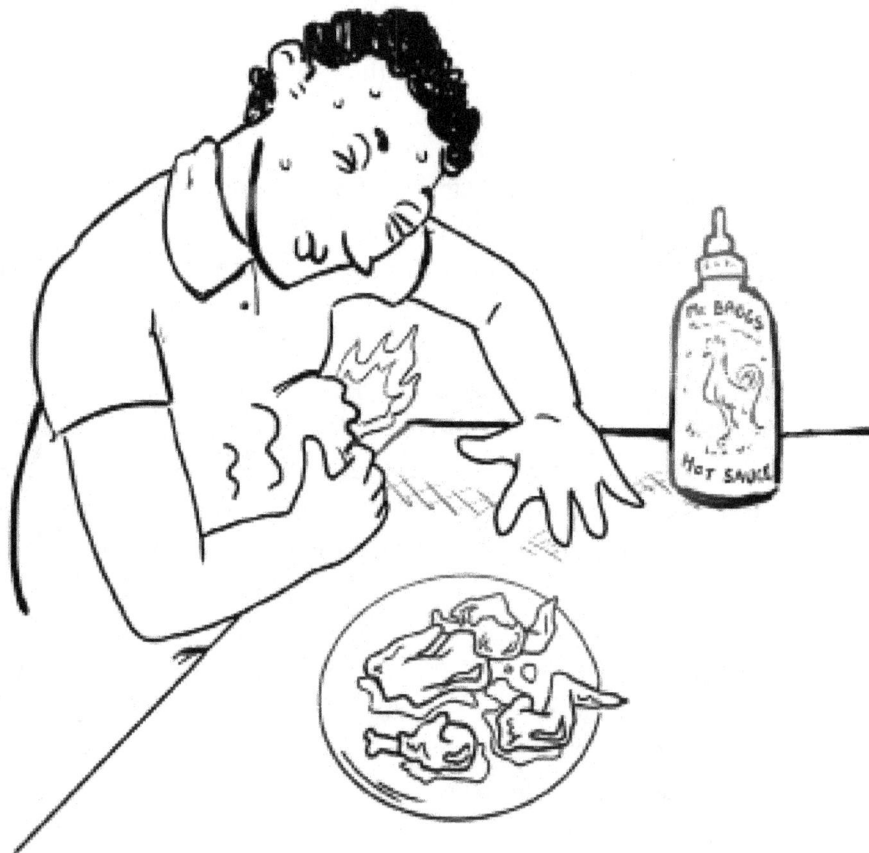

"I Have a Love-Hate Relationship with Spicy Wings."

MYTH Peptic Ulcers Are Caused by Eating Acidic and Spicy Foods

TRUTH Acidic and Spicy Foods Don't Cause Peptic Ulcers

PEPTIC ULCERS CAN'T BE BLAMED on spicy or acidic foods. If you've already got an ulcer, yes, spicy foods can worsen some of the symptoms, like abdominal pain. But the truth is, 90 percent of peptic ulcers are caused by the bacterium *Helicobater pylori* (*H. pylori*). *H. pylori* infection can be diagnosed with a blood test, a breath test, or an endoscopy. Rarely, a bleeding ulcer can become life threatening, but most of the time the condition can be successfully treated in about two weeks with a course of prescription antibiotics to combat the bacterium.

H. pylori was first discovered in the stomachs of patients with gastritis and ulcers in 1982 by Drs. Barry Marshall and Robin Warren of Perth in western Australia. At the time, researchers didn't believe that any bacteria could live in the acidic environment of the human stomach. The story goes that Dr. Marshall decided to prove that a bacterium caused ulcers by ingesting a slurry of the bacteria and performing an endoscopy on himself. He and his fellow researcher later received the Nobel Prize in physiology for their work.

According to the Centers for Disease Control and Prevention (CDC), "Approximately 25 million Americans will have an ulcer at some point in their lifetime. People of any age can get an ulcer and women are affected just as often as men. There are approximately 500,000 –850,000 new cases of ulcer disease each year and more than 1 million ulcer-related hospitalizations each year."

Though spicy foods aren't to blame, some things we ingest *can* contribute to the formation of ulcers. In about 10 percent of cases, it has been shown that the regular use of painkillers and other types of drugs led to the formation of a patient's ulcer. It's actually an all-too-frequent occurrence in elderly patients who take a lot of ibuprofen (a nonsteroidal anti-inflammatory drug or NSAID) for chronic pain.

Researchers are trying to develop a vaccine to prevent ulcers, but are still trying to figure out how the bacterium is transmitted. For now, here are a few research-based facts on how to avoid an ulcer:

- Don't smoke. Heavy smokers are more likely to develop certain types of ulcers than nonsmokers.
- Drink alcohol moderately. Heavy consumption of alcohol has been shown to contribute to the development of ulcers.
- Don't overuse painkillers.

For those patients in my practice who do develop an ulcer and test positive for the bacterium, I recommend a 10 to 14-day course of antibiotics. For most people, that does the trick. There's no need to stop enjoying that spicy Sriracha dressing or an occasional glass of red wine. Enjoy. Cheers!

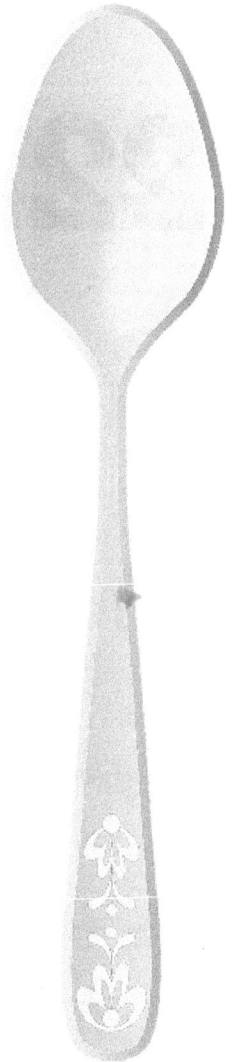

"90 percent of peptic ulcers are caused by the bacterium Helicobacter pylori (H. pylori)."

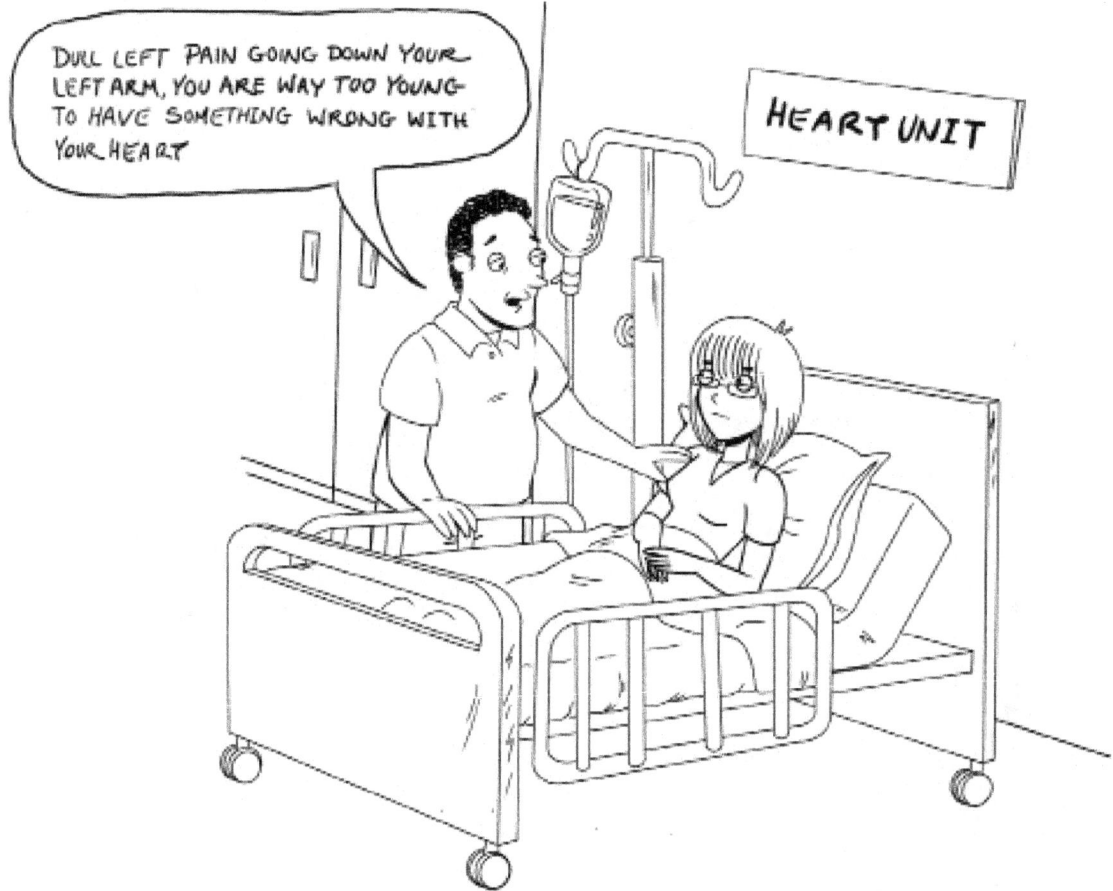

"Young Women Don't Have Heart Attacks, Right?"

23

MYTH Heart Disease and Strokes Are an "Old Man's Disease"

TRUTH Heart Disease and Strokes Are Suffered by Young People, Too

The older you get, the more things wear out, the more clogged your arteries get, the less you tend to exercise, and so on. After a while, our age just starts catching up with us. That's why old people end up suffering heart attacks and strokes. Sound familiar? That's the story we like to tell ourselves–that heart disease is an "old man's disease." Sadly, that's just not true anymore.

It's a mistake–and for some people, a dangerous one–to believe that only the old are afflicted. A study of 28,000 people hospitalized for heart attacks from 1995 to 2014 was recently published in the American Heart Association's journal, *Circulation*. It showed 30 percent of those patients were young, age 35 to 54. "More importantly," as reported on heart.org, "they found the people having heart attacks were increasingly young, from 27 percent at the start of the study to 32 percent at the end. Cardiac disease is sometimes considered an old man's disease, but the trajectory of heart attacks among young people is going the wrong way."

Researchers are still trying to figure out why so many young people, especially young women, are now suffering from heart disease. It could be that they have one or more of the known risk factors, which include smoking, alcohol and drug abuse; a family history of heart disease; genetically high cholesterol; and certain other inherited traits. Many of these factors are either detectable or traceable in a patient's family history.

If you suspect that you might have one or more of these risk factors, whatever your age, you should seek out your physician's advice about how to anticipate and deal with any health problems that might arise. With a few simple tests, your doctor might uncover something that you've overlooked. For example, your doctor could perform a test for low-density lipo-protein (LDL), a type of cholesterol found in the body. If the doctor discovers that you have an LDL-reading of 200 (the normal range is 100), he or she might suggest some changes. One meeting with your doctor could reveal a problem in your body that might ultimately cause a heart attack or stroke at a young age. Wouldn't you like the opportunity to address such an issue early and potentially avoid a life-threatening scenario?

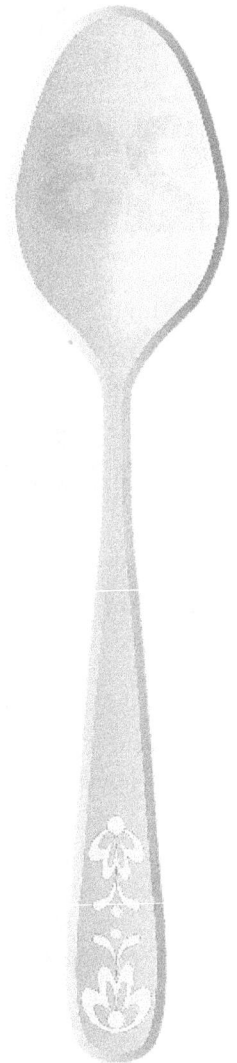

"One meeting with your doctor could reveal a problem in your body that might ultimately cause a heart attack or stroke at a young age."

"Houston, We Have a Problem!"

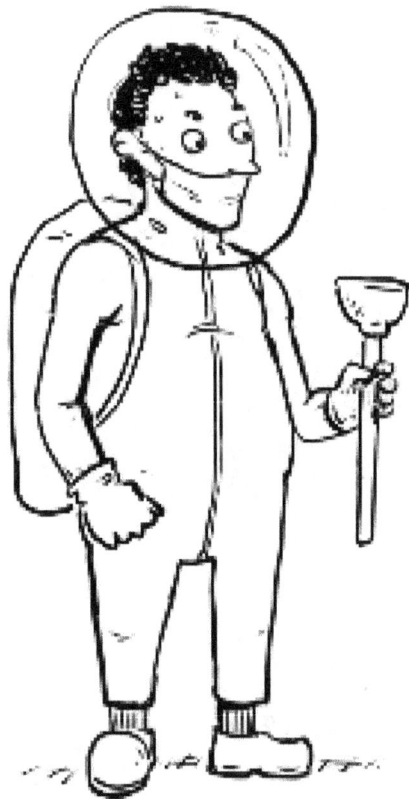

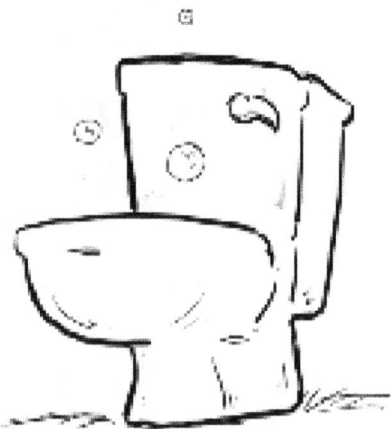

24

MYTH You Can Catch an STD from a Toilet

TRUTH STDs Are Not Transmitted by Toilet Seats

THERE'S NO QUESTION THAT THE TOILET seats in most (read "all") public restrooms, and actually many household bathrooms, are playgrounds for the viruses and bacteria that cause sexually transmitted diseases (STDs). Yes, you can find the makings of chlamydia, gonorrhea, herpes, syphilis, and genital warts on millions of toilet seats. However, the germs that cause these diseases remain alive for only a very short time after they've landed on a toilet seat, often for no more than a minute or two. Moreover, in order for you to get infected, the germs would have to somehow move from the toilet seat to the inside of your urethral or genital tract. The only other route would be for them to enter your bloodstream. Perhaps, in the most unlikely of cases, you could contract a disease by sitting on a still-living cluster of germs with a cut or open sore on your buttocks, thighs, or scrotum. It's possible, but extremely unlikely. "To my knowledge," says Abigail Salyers, president of the American Society for Microbiology, "no one has ever acquired an STD from a toilet seat—unless they were having sex on [one]!"

This isn't to say that you shouldn't protect yourself from STDs by practicing safe sex. In fact, STDs threaten millions of Americans and are on the rise—and not from toilet seats. According to the CDC, there were a total of 2,295,739 STD cases in the United States in 2017, a record high. And the consequences can be quite serious. The CDC reports that "Chlamydia is the most commonly reported STD, with approximately 1.7 million cases reported in 2017. Young women (ages 15-24) account for nearly half (45 percent) of reported cases and face the most severe consequences of an undiagnosed infection. Untreated STDs, like chlamydia and gonorrhea, put women at increased risk for pelvic inflammatory disease which may result in chronic pelvic pain, infertility, and potentially a life-threatening ectopic pregnancy.

It is estimated that undiagnosed STDs cause infertility in more than 20,000 women each year." That is a sobering statistic.

Many people are too embarrassed to ask their doctor for an STD test. Don't be. I give my patients an STD test with no questions asked. I do, however, take the time to explain to my patients that it is mature and healthy to use protection during sex and sexual partners should always respect your right to have protection. STDs are a significant health problem, so it's important to concentrate on the real cause: unprotected sex, not unclean toilet seats.

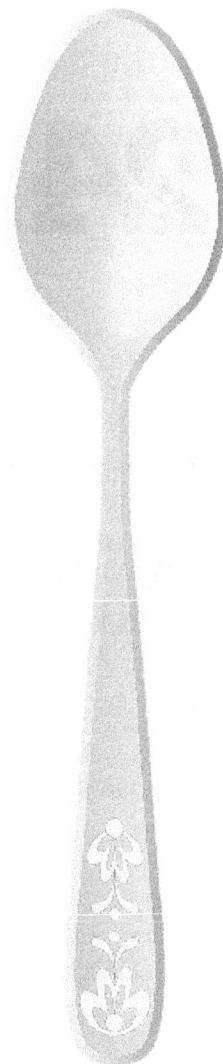

"The germs that cause these diseases remain alive for only a very short time."

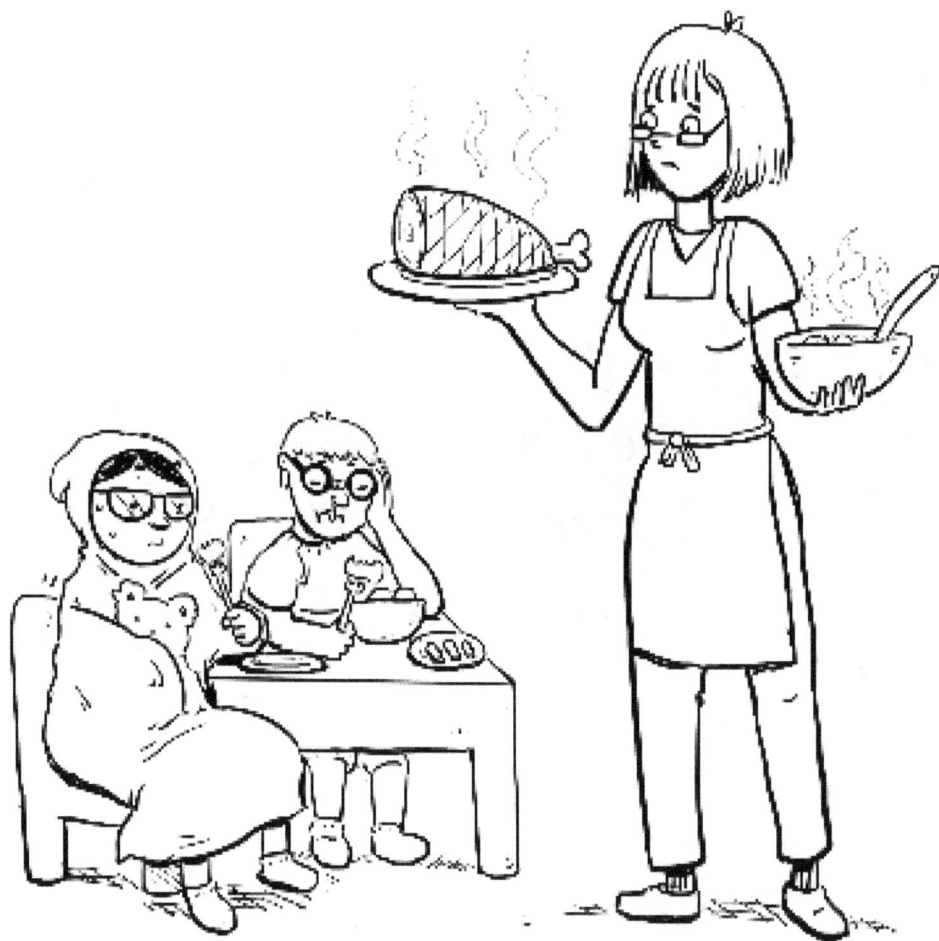

"Is It Feed a Cold or Starve a Cold?"

25

MYTH Feed a Cold and Starve a Fever

TRUTH Feed a Cold and Feed a Fever Because Sick or Well our Bodies Always Need Energy

NO ONE KNOWS EXACTLY WHERE this myth came from, but boy did it stick! In a 1574 dictionary by John Withals, it was noted that "fasting is a great remedy of fever." The idea was based on the belief that eating food would help the body generate warmth during a cold virus while avoiding food could cool it down when overheated by a fever. This might have made perfect sense before modern science was able to study such correlations. Today, science tells a different story.

But think about it, how many times have you heard this phrase in your life. "Feed a cold and starve a fever" is practically a national mantra for the sick. Yet, from my point of view as a doctor, it makes no sense at all! *Scientific American* said it best when it offered that the saying should actually be: "Feed a cold *and* feed a fever." Why? Because when your body's dealing with illness of any kind, it needs energy. Where do humans find energy? In food, primarily. So why would you starve yourself when your body needs energy to heal?

When you've got a fever, your body's immune system is working overtime to combat some germ to which you were exposed. One consequence of that internal combat is an increased metabolism, which means you need more energy than usual, not less. Even if you've lost your appetite as a result of your illness, you should try to keep some fuel in the furnace to help your body manage the war going on within.

But the plot thickens. It might be important what type of food you feed your cold and fever based on what type of illness you have. Science has begun looking into this topic.

A study published in *Cell* led by Ruslan Medzhitov, an immunologist at Yale University, sought to explore whether the age-old adage had any truth behind it. He and his colleagues conducted a study on mice by infecting them with either a bacterium that causes food poisoning or one that causes the flu virus. They force-fed half the mice pure glucose. After 10 days all the bacteria-infected mice who had continued being fed had died, while more than half that had naturally avoided food during their illness lived.

For the mice infected with the flu, it was the opposite. More than 75 percent of the force-fed mice lived, while only about 10 percent lived if they hadn't. Food was protective against the virus, but detrimental to the bacterial infection. As Medzhitov told statnews.com, "To our complete surprise, we found that force feeding was protective" in viral infections. Intrigued, the team conducted more experiments, and found that glucose, but not proteins or fats, was the dangerous component of foods during a bacterial infection. A similar 2002 study of humans, which was published in the *American Society for Microbiology*, reached a similar conclusion.

There's still much more research to be done, but here's my two cents on the topic: Okay, I get it, you feel awful. I visit patients in the hospital when they have pneumonia or other infections. They lack the motivation to eat or drink anything. I tell them they have to eat something because they need energy. In these cases, food is a sort of medicine.

There's one thing I know for sure: fevers dehydrate us. We typically don't want to eat because we feel lousy (and we can't smell our food because we're congested). But fevers do increase our desire for fluid, which fills us up a bit. There is stuff in our mucus that helps us fight bacteria and viruses in our respiratory passages when we have a cold. Hydration helps with mucous production. So even if you choose to skip the feeding part, you definitely want to stay hydrated. The hot vapor from warm liquids such as tea or soup also help to keep the mucus flowing. That's why mom's chicken soup is one home remedy I *do* believe in. Eat it when you're sick. It will hydrate your system and provide important protein.

My patients tell me about all their home remedies. I always find it fascinating to discover where they heard about them. Usually, it was a parent who shared the home remedy. Sometimes, though, a relative or knowledgeable family member has passed down the

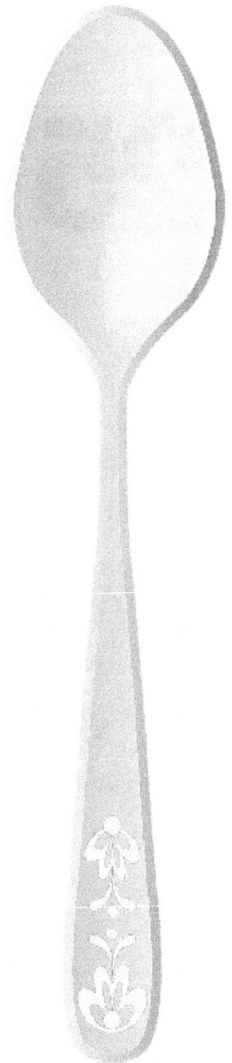

remedy. Some home remedies have been handed down in families for generations. Most of the time, these remedies were imparted in a spirit of love and caring. I think this is one reason why they work. Love and caring do have healing powers. That's not a myth. There is scientific evidence to support this statement. So the next time you offer your homemade chicken soup to a family member, remind him or her it's not "Feed a cold and starve a fever." Rather, it's "Feed a cold *and* feed a fever!"

"I Tried, But I Just Can't Stop Cracking my Knuckles!"

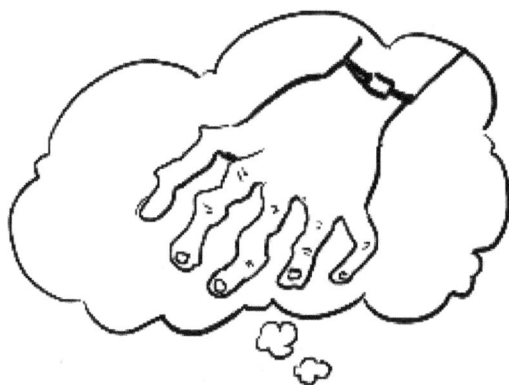

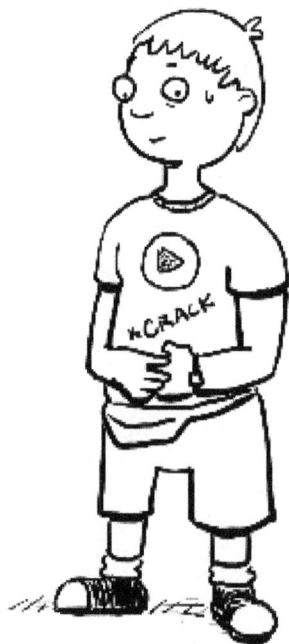

26

MYTH Cracking Your Knuckles Causes Arthritis

TRUTH Knuckle Cracking Is Annoying, Not Dangerous

DESPITE WHAT YOUR MOTHER TOLD you for your *entire* childhood, cracking your knuckles does not cause arthritis and appears to have no harmful side effects. Believe it or not, there have been a number of studies looking at this issue.

According to a study published in the *Western Journal of Medicine*, "A survey of a geriatric patient population with a history of knuckle cracking failed to show a correlation between knuckle cracking and degenerative changes of the metacarpal phalangeal joints."

Another study published in the *Annals of Rheumatic Diseases* studied another, larger group of people and came to a similar conclusion: the study found no correlation between knuckle cracking and arthritis.

Interesting aside. That "pop" sound you hear when you crack your knuckles has also been studied. According to the Harvard Medical School: "Cracking your knuckles may aggravate the people around you, but it probably won't raise your risk for arthritis. The 'pop' of a cracked knuckle is actually caused by bubbles bursting in the synovial fluid–the fluid that helps lubricate joints. The bubbles pop when you pull the bones apart, either by stretching the fingers or bending them backward, creating negative pressure."

One study did reveal that habitual knuckle-crackers are more likely to develop swollen hands and reduced grip strength. For those of you annoyed by the knuckle-crackers, you might have to resort to this possibility in order to discourage them because the "Cracking your knuckles causes arthritis" tattle no longer appears to hold water.

"I'm Not Making THAT Sacrifice for Beauty!"

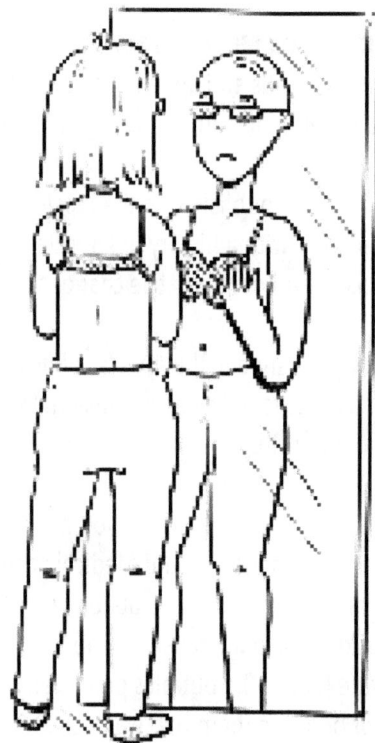

27

MYTH Wearing an Underwire Bra Causes Breast Cancer

TRUTH Underwire Bras Do Not Cause Breast Cancer

Sometimes fear–in this case fear of breast cancer–causes us to look for ways to control things over which we have little control. That's one theory posited in *Dr. Susan Love's Breast Book* to explain the persistent myth that wearing an underwire bra causes breast cancer.

The idea that bras may cause cancer was fueled by the 1995 book *Dressed to Kill* by Sydney Ross Singer and Soma Grismaijer. The book claimed that women who wear underwire bras for 12 hours a day have a much higher risk of developing breast cancer than women who do not wear bras. The authors maintained that bras restrict the lymph system, which result in a build-up of toxins in the breasts. There has never been any scientific evidence to support this claim.

In fact, studies published on the subject have found the opposite. In one study, researchers interviewed postmenopausal female participants about their lifetime bra-wearing patterns. "Evaluating more than 1,000 women with breast cancer and almost 500 who did not have breast cancer, the researchers found no evidence of a connection between the number of hours spent wearing a bra or wearing an underwire bra and increased breast cancer risk."

According to the National Center for Health Research, a woman has a 12.1 percent chance of being diagnosed with breast cancer in her lifetime. Unfortunately, that's no myth. Here are seven scientifically-validated risk factors for breast cancer:

- **Your Sex:** Women represent 99 percent of all breast cancer patients

- **Your Age:** About 65 percent of women are over 55 years old when they are diagnosed.
- **Your Race.** After age 45, white women are more likely to get breast cancer than black women, but black women have a higher incidence before age 45 and are more likely to die from it.
- **Your Family History.** Certain inherited gene mutations (BRCA1 and BRCA2) increase the risk of developing breast cancer. Genetic testing may benefit you. Consult your doctor.
- **Beginning Menstruation Early.** If you began menstruating before age 12, you are at an increased risk of breast cancer.
- **Starting Menopause Late (after age 55).** If you start menopause late, you face a higher risk of breast cancer.
- **Dense Breast Tissue (including fibrocystic breasts).** This condition can increase the risk of breast cancer

It is a good idea for women to do monthly self-examinations of their breasts and also schedule annual wellness visits with their doctor for all of their screenings. Almost all insurance plans now cover breast-cancer screening. Based on past test results and other factors, the initial or follow-up tests may be an ultrasound or diagnostic mammogram, rather than a screening mammogram.

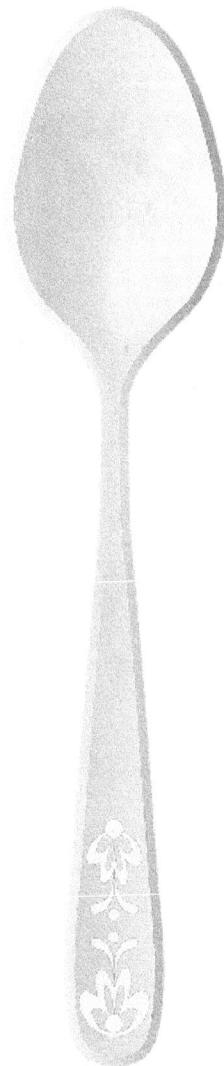

"Researchers found no evidence of a connection between the number of hours spent wearing an underwire bra and increased breast cancer risk."

"Honey, I'm Worried."

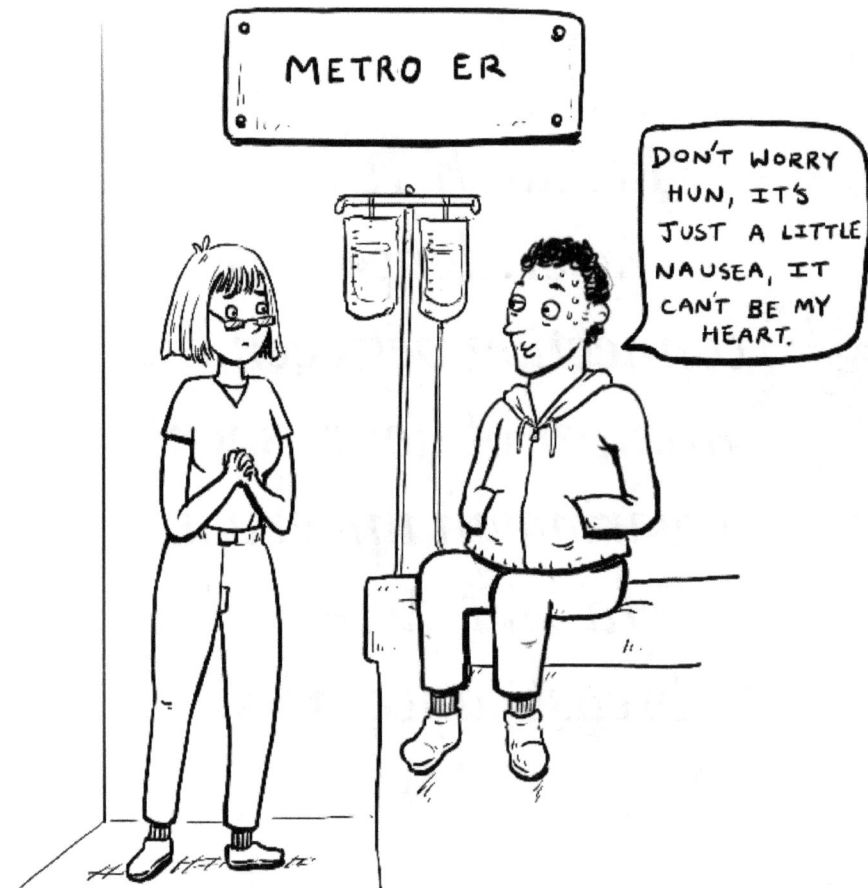

28

MYTH Heart Attacks Are Always Preceded by Chest Pain

TRUTH Other Symptoms in Addition to Chest Pain Can Precede a Heart Attack

WHILE IT'S TRUE THAT HEART ATTACKS—in both men and women—are commonly preceded by a feeling of fullness, squeezing, or pressure in the chest area, pain is not always present. It is most of the time, but not all of the time. There are other signs and symptoms of impending heart trouble of which you should be aware, especially if two or more are present:

- Pain or discomfort in one or both arms, the back, neck, jaw or stomach
- Shortness of breath with or without chest discomfort
- Cold sweat, nausea or lightheadedness

And just to make diagnosing your symptoms a bit more challenging, 45 percent of all heart attacks in the United States are silent, which means they are completely without symptoms. Diabetics are at the highest risk of these atypical presentations. Men and women present differently before a heart attack, with women more likely to experience shortness of breath, nausea and/or vomiting, and back or jaw pain. The other thing to remember about chest pain is that it could indicate other serious problems such as pneumonia or a blood clot in your lung.

If you have chest pain or any of the symptoms listed above, it's better to go directly to a hospital emergency room (ER), rather than an urgent or immediate care center. Time is of the essence. And if your chest pain is serious, the urgent- or immediate-care center will simply refer you to the ER anyway, so it's best to just go there directly.

When you arrive at the ER, the doctor will ask you about your past medical history and the exact nature of your chest pain. He or she may order an electrocardiogram (EKG) and possibly a heart echo test. It is a test that measures the electrical activity of the heartbeat. The heart echo test, or echocardiogram, uses high frequency sound waves (ultrasound) to create pictures of your heart. The test is also called echocardiography or diagnostic cardiac ultrasound.

Keep in mind that both EKGs and heart echo tests can be wrong. The patient's history is one of the most important diagnostic tools for determining whether the chest pain is signaling a possible heart attack.

The risk factors for heart attack are high blood pressure, diabetes, high cholesterol, smoking and family history. As a doctor, I am especially worried about my diabetic patients. They are at a higher risk of heart disease. I can remember one patient who came to me with weakness and nausea. We went ahead and ordered an EKG and found out that she was having a mild heart attack. Because we caught it early, she was able to be treated at the hospital and released with no long-term damage. She's doing quite well several years out. As this case shows, diabetics often have atypical heart attack symptoms.

More important than the signs of a heart attack, are the actions you can take to lower your risk of developing heart disease and suffering from a heart attack. The US National Library of Medicine lists these ten actions you can take:

- Control your blood pressure
- Keep your cholesterol and triglyceride levels under control
- Stay at a healthy weight
- Eat a healthy diet
- Get regular exercise
- Limit your alcohol intake
- Do not smoke
- Manage your stress
- Manage Diabetes, if you have it
- Make sure to get enough sleep

Because the myth that heart attacks are always preceded by chest pain remains so popular, people tend to dismiss other possible warning signs. Don't be one of those people. Listen to your body and either call your doctor or dial 911. Don't let this myth put your life at risk.

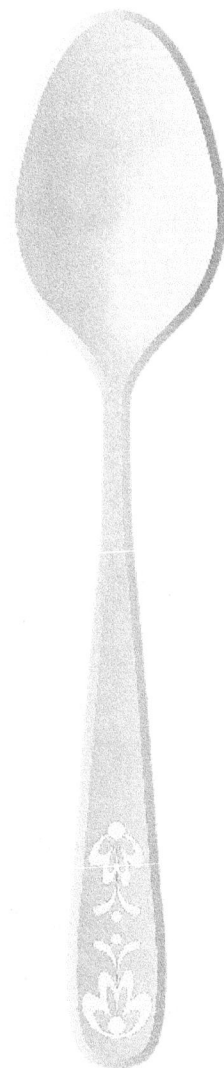

"45 percent of all heart attacks in the U.S. are silent or completely without symptoms."

"There's Nothing Wrong With a Little Extra Ice Cream!"

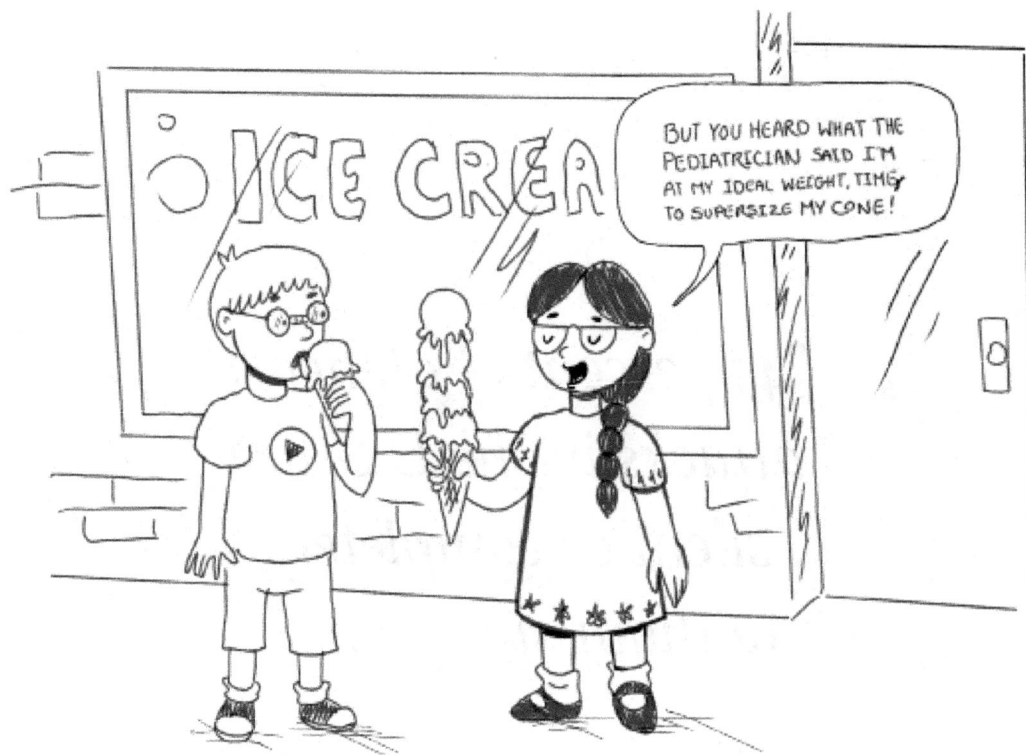

29

MYTH Only Overweight People Develop Type 2 Diabetes

TRUTH Many People of Average Weight Develop Type 2 Diabetes

ACCORDING TO THE AMERICAN DIABETES ASSOCIATION, being overweight is one risk factor for Diabetes 2, "but other risk factors such as how much physical activity you get, family history, ethnicity, and age also play a role. Unfortunately, many people think that weight is the only risk factor for type 2 diabetes, but many people with type 2 diabetes are at a normal weight or only moderately overweight." In fact, only 30 percent of overweight people develop type 2 diabetes.

Type 2 diabetes is a chronic and progressive condition that impacts the way your body controls the amount of sugar (glucose) in the blood. Insulin is a hormone that transfers glucose from the blood into cells to produce the energy needed for daily activities. In people who have type 2 diabetes, insulin can't do its job. That's because too little insulin is produced to keep glucose levels normal, or the body fails to respond to it. Glucose builds up in the blood when you are insulin resistant, leading to the symptoms associated with type 2 diabetes.

Genetics and lifestyle choices are the most common causes of the disease. According to EndocrineWeb.com, "The medical community is hard at work trying to figure out the certain genetic mutations that lead to a risk of type 2...but lifestyle choices are also important. You can, for example, have a genetic mutation that *may* make you susceptible to type 2, but if you take good care of your body, you may not develop diabetes."

When a young 20 or 30-year-old comes into my office and tells me about eating a lot of sweets or junk food, I immediately screen for prediabetes, even if he or she is of an average weight. Unfortunately, I find that many of them, especially those that have not been to a doctor in years, already have full-blown diabetes.

Remember, people of all body types develop diabetes. Left untreated, type 2 diabetes can cause a heart attack or stroke. It can lead to blindness, circulatory problems, kidney failure and a host of other unpleasant and life-altering consequences. That's why it's important to have a strong relationship with your primary care doctor and have him or her conduct annual, age-specific screenings for diabetes.

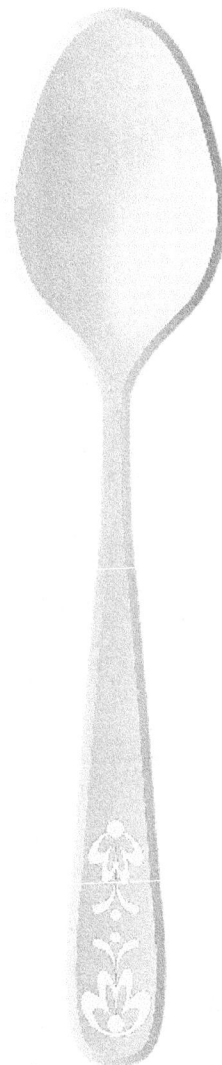

"When a young adult comes into my office and tells me about eating a lot of sweets or junk food, I screen for pre-diabetes."

"Buy Organic or Swell Up Like a Balloon!"

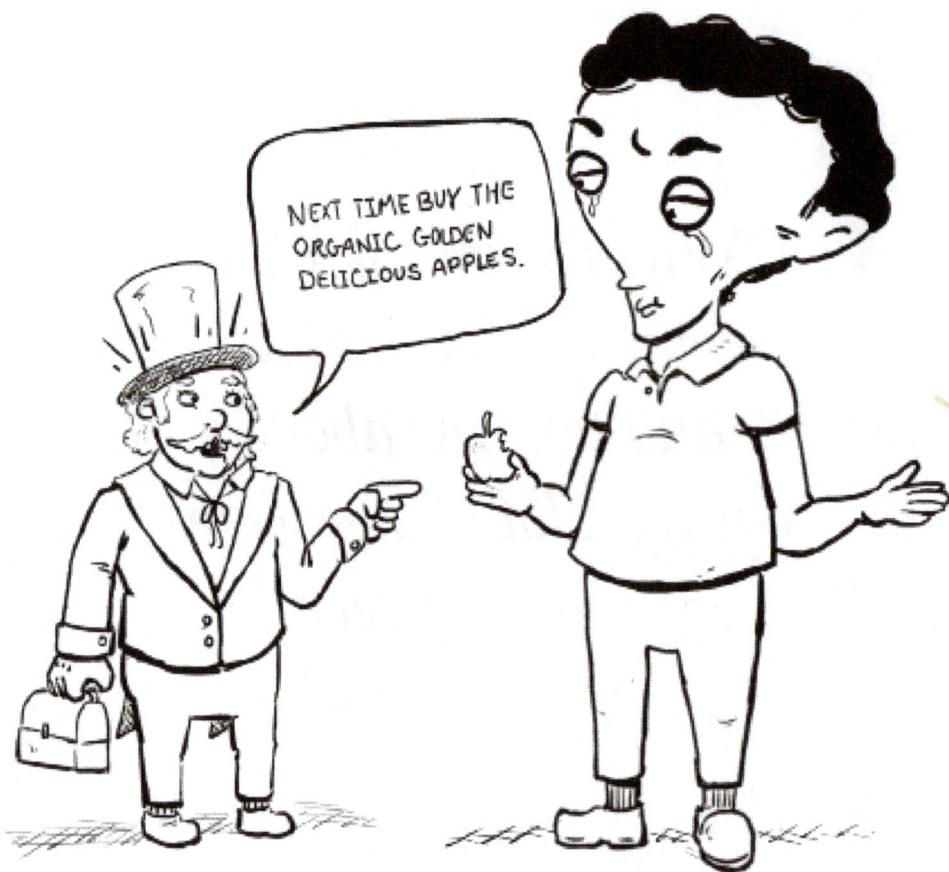

30

MYTH Organic Foods Are Hypoallergenic

TRUTH Organic Foods Can Contain Allergens

AS I SAID EARLIER IN THIS BOOK, food labeling is a complex business here in the good 'ole USA. Oversight of the use of the term "organic" on a food product label starts at the US Department of Agriculture (USDA). The USDA has actually designated four levels of organic labeling: "100 percent organic" (gets a USDA seal), "organic" (also gets a USDA seal), "Made with Organic" (no seal) and "Organic Ingredients" (no seal). Trouble is, not one of these levels mentions that the product must be hypoallergenic in order to be labeled as organic.

The label "hypoallergenic," which means a product is unlikely to cause an allergic reaction, can be extremely important if you have a child that reacts to certain substances. Baby formula that is labeled hypoallergenic typically does not contain milk protein, which can trigger reactions in lactose-intolerant children. In the case of a true food allergy, a labeling mistake can even be fatal in some situations. Unfortunately, just because something is labeled hypoallergenic, doesn't mean that it can't cause an allergic reaction in some people.

Rarely will you see the terms organic and hypoallergenic on the same product label, and never assume when you see one that it also implies the other. It does not. If the food you want to eat needs to be organic *and* hypoallergenic then both labels must be present on the packaging...and even *that* doesn't imply complete safety. While food labeling has some benefits for consumers, don't fool yourself, it is a highly charged, highly politicized field, influenced by big lobbies with big money.

The bottom line is that people with food allergies or serious sensitivities need to read and understand the labels on the foods they consume. It's not safe to have a general understanding of a labeling term. If you have a question about a food's ingredients, you should call the manufacturer. There's too much at stake to rely on the vagueness and lack of clarity in a food label.

"Oh, No! Did We Get Too Close?"

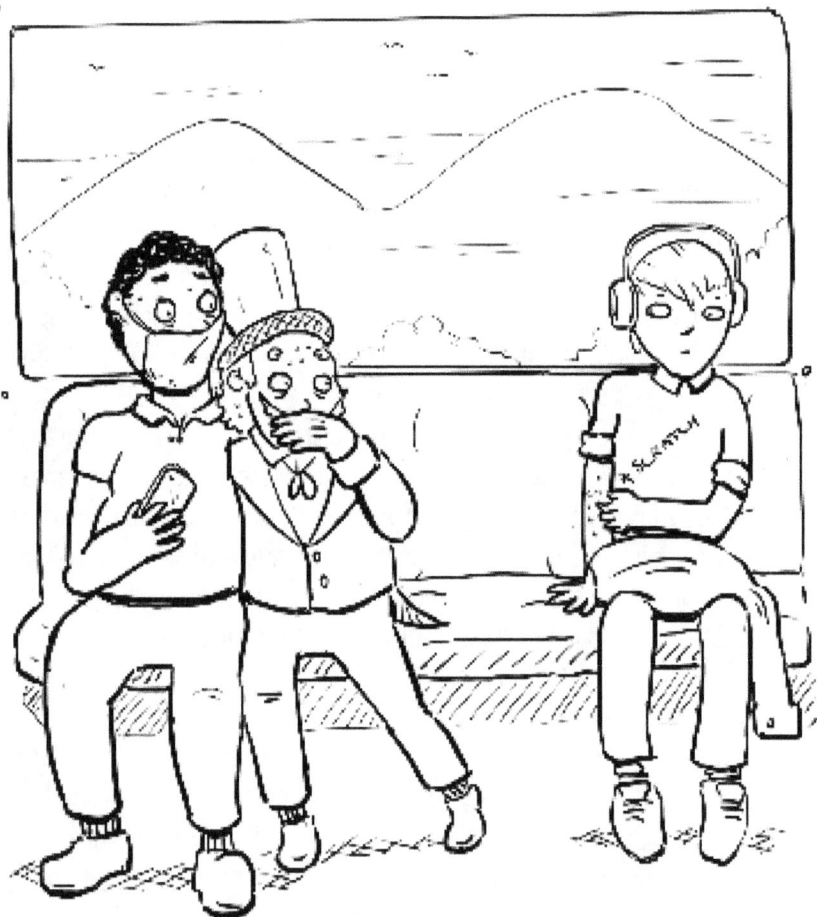

31

MYTH Psoriasis Is a Contagious Skin Condition
TRUTH Psoriasis Is a Noncontagious Autoimmune Disease

Psoriasis is actually an autoimmune disease that impacts the skin. As such, it's not a contagious disease that can be spread through any kind of physical contact. Unfortunately, as with so many autoimmune diseases, no cure has yet been found. The good news, however, is a number of medications and topical treatments have proven to be very effective in moderating the disease's appearance and reversing some of its symptoms.

According to psoriasis.com, "When you have psoriasis, your immune system is overactive. This creates inflammation inside the body, which is a cause of the symptoms you see on the skin. More healthy cells are produced than normal. Those excess cells get pushed to the surface of your skin too quickly. Normally, it takes about a month for your skin cells to cycle through your body. With psoriasis, it takes days. Your body simply can't shed skin cells that quickly, so the cells build up on the surface of your skin. The thick, red patches you see on your skin (called plaques) are actually a buildup of excess skin cells."

So, just to dispel another myth about psoriasis, the **appearance of those red patches has nothing to do with hygiene. It's all about your genes.** "One out of 3 people with psoriasis reports having a relative with the disease," psoriasis.com reports. "And researchers say that up to 10 percent of the general population may inherit one or more genes that predispose them to psoriasis, though only 2 to 3 percent of people with the gene actually develop the disease." Certain environmental factors are thought to trigger the psoriasis genes, such as stress: skin injuries like cuts, scrapes and bug bites: infections like strep throat or rush; and certain medications.

I see a lot of patients with mild to moderate cases of psoriasis. They can typically be treated with topical steroids or topical Vitamin A derivatives. When a case is more severe, I refer my patients to a dermatologist, who may prescribe light therapy or methotrexate or cyclosporin. It is a good idea to see your primary care doctor first, so he or she can assess your overall health before referring you to a specialist.

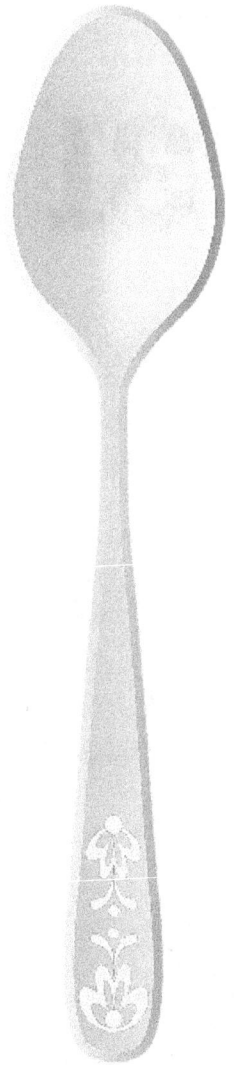

"Psoriasis is an autoimmune disease. It is not contagious."

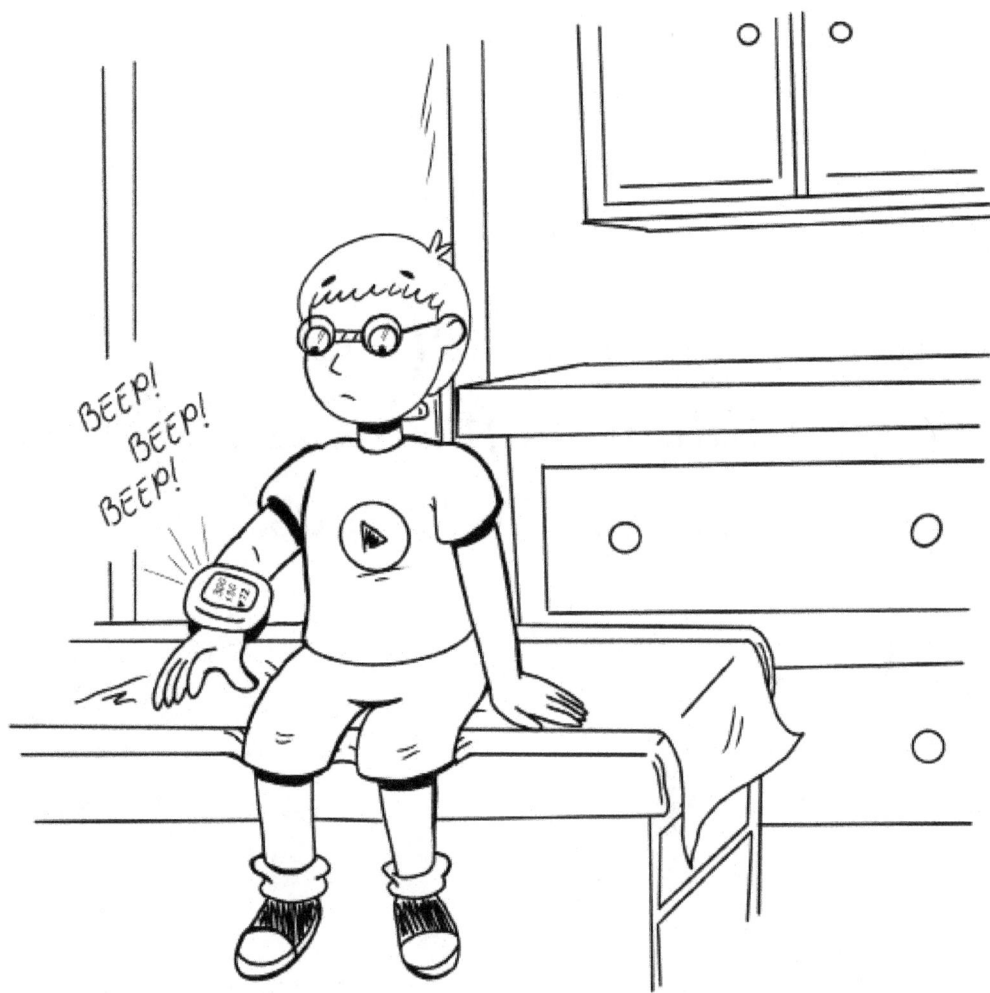

32

MYTH High Blood Pressure Is an Old-Age Disease

TRUTH Hypertension Can Be a Silent Killer at Any Age

HIGH BLOOD PRESSURE, ALSO CALLED HYPERTENSION, is known as the "silent killer" because it can be asymptomatic for so long. It impacts 1 in 3 adults, which is about 75 million people. Now, research by the National Institutes of Health suggests that 19 percent of young adults have high blood pressure, indicating a higher risk for young adults than previously believed.

Hypertension is a dangerous disease that can cause heart attacks and strokes, if left untreated. Dr. Wanpen Vongpatanasin, who headed up the largest study looking at a condition known as isolated systolic hypertension (ISH) in young adults, says "the increased prevalence of traditional risk factors in the young, including obesity, diabetes mellitus, and renal disease, increases the risk of developing hypertension in younger adults."

Yes, there's a significant genetic (familial) component in the development of hypertension, and so it does, in a sense, "run in families." However, wise lifestyle choices (diet, exercise, regular health screening) can often prevent its occurrence entirely, even in those with a family history of the disease. In truth, hypertension is more of a genetic and lifestyle disease than it is an old-age disease.

A recent large study revealed that many young adults in their twenties and thirties prefer telemedicine and urgent care to visiting their primary care physician. The problem is that blood pressure isn't often taken in telemedicine situations and urgent care facilities are not an ideal place to look for underlying health risks like high blood pressure. If you go this route, it is to your advantage to follow up with an experienced primary care doctor who can spot trends in your blood pressure and recommend lifestyle changes, such as a low-salt diet and more exercise. These measures can help keep blood pressure in check and prevent the need for medications.

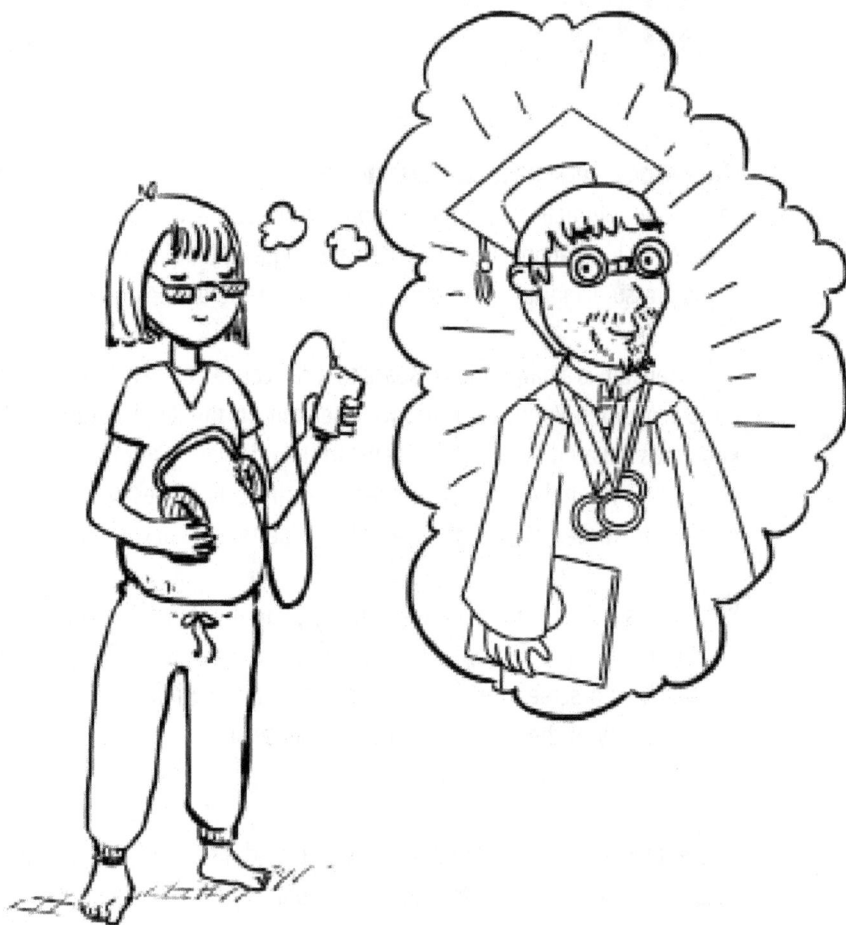

"Amadeus, Amadeus, Do Your Magic and Make Me Proud!"

33

MYTH Playing Mozart While Pregnant Makes a Smarter Baby

TRUTH Mozart is a Stirring Classic, But Won't Make Your Baby Smarter

EVERYONE KNOWS ABOUT THE "MOZART EFFECT," right? It received so much press attention that it started a national craze. Hundreds of products were created based on the belief that listening to Mozart would make people smarter, especially kids. The idea that babies in utero would be smarter if they listened to classical music emerged from this hype. In fact, one year, the governor of Georgia mandated that a classical music CD containing a Mozart sonata be given to all new babies when they left a state hospital. Despite all the hype, the Mozart Effect is not real. According to an article in *Psychology Today*, "Researchers at the University of Vienna (Pietschnig, Voracek, & Formann, 2010) performed a meta-analysis of nearly 40 studies. Guess what? *They found no evidence that listening to Mozart's music 'enhanced' cognitive abilities in any way.*"

There's nothing wrong with playing classical music for your child, either before or after he or she is born. However, don't expect your child to turn into a genius as a result. There are many things that contribute to a child's cognitive development in utero and out. If you want your child to get off to a good start, support a healthy pregnancy by eating a healthy diet, enjoying moderate exercise and avoiding anything that could hinder your baby's development, such as drugs, alcohol, tobacco and caffeine.

I do not treat children in my practice, but understand from research that at four months, a child in utero has fairly well developed hearing and by six months starts to turn its head toward voices in the womb. In the last three months of pregnancy, in utero babies even start to recognize some repeated words. Studies show that deeper, lower sounds are easier for them to make out. So, if you are not into classical music, that is okay! Just put on your favorite tunes and maybe your baby will learn to love your music as much as you do.

"I've Heard Rumors That Chemo Is Worse Than Cancer!"

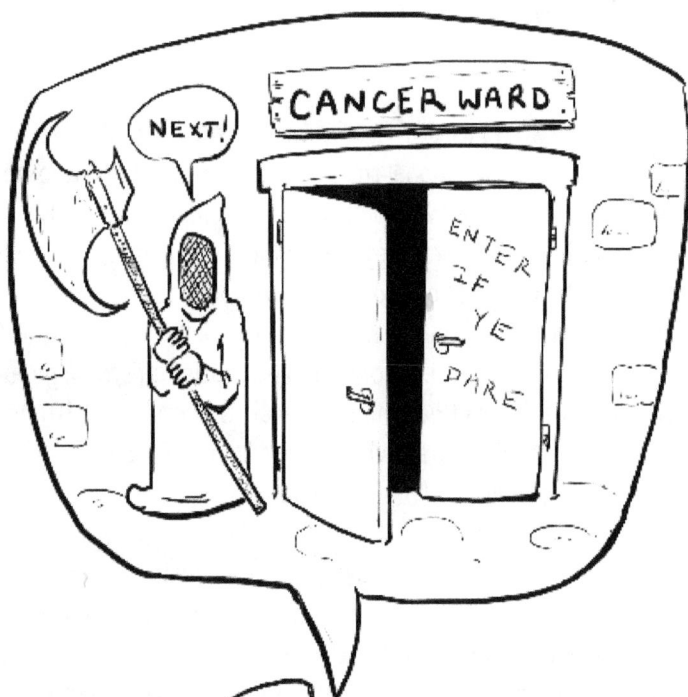

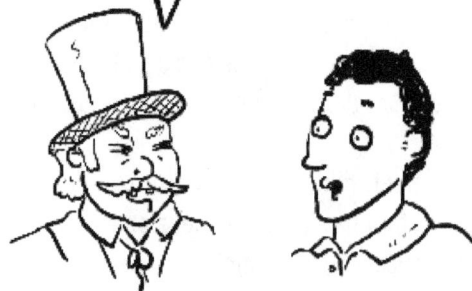

34

MYTH Cancer Treatments Kill More People Than They Cure

TRUTH Cancer Treatment Side Effects Are Not Worse Than Their Ability To Cure

IT'S TRUE TODAY THAT MORE PEOPLE are still dying of cancer (in all its forms) than are being cured. It is also true that some people die during or right after their cancer treatment. These are the tough realities that researchers, doctors and patients face every day in their battle to find answers and cures.

Cancer treatments, even when successful, often have toxic and unpleasant side effects like hair loss, nausea, or vomiting. But people who believe cancer treatments lead to death are mistaken. It's the cancer and the patient's compromised immune system caused by the ongoing battle with cancer that ultimately kill. It is a fatal one-two punch.

Many medical treatments have side effects. The two main treatments for cancer–chemotherapy and radiation therapy–are no exception. The question is whether the side effects are worth the potential benefit. If you have breast cancer and it has been detected early, surgery to remove the tumor, followed by chemo and/or radiation therapies, could put the breast cancer into remission and extend your life significantly. However, if your breast cancer is advanced and the prognosis is poor, perhaps putting your body through treatment isn't worth it. Maybe you would rather spend your last months of life enjoying experiences with your family and friends, rather than undergoing treatment in a hospital. These are the types of difficult cost-versus-benefit discussions patients must have with their doctors when cancer strikes.

Cancer is still a leading cause of death across the globe. According to the World Health Organization, nearly 1 in 6 deaths worldwide are due to cancer. But new treatment options and medical advances have improved the prognosis for many cancer patients over the past few decades. Researchers and doctors are making significant progress in creating chemo-therapy and other treatment regimens with lower toxicity and fewer side effects.

Slowly but surely, the medical community is making progress and providing new treatment regimens that are highly successful in combating specific types of cancer. And more good news: The survival rate in the United States is very high for many types of cancer. Breast cancer has the highest cure rate, followed by prostate, testicular, thyroid, melanoma, cervical, and Hodgkin's lymphoma. If these are caught before Stage II, there is a 90 percent, five-year remission rate and most likely a cure. Much work remains, but progress is being made. If you are diagnosed with cancer, talk to your doctor with an open mind about your treatment options.

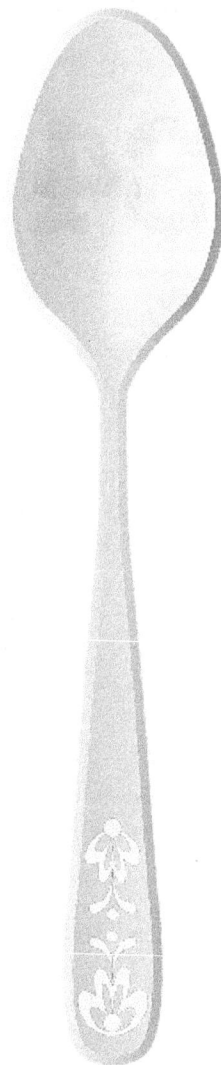

"The survival rate in the United States is very high for many types of cancer."

"Yeah, So It's Like Putting a Garden Hose Up There!"

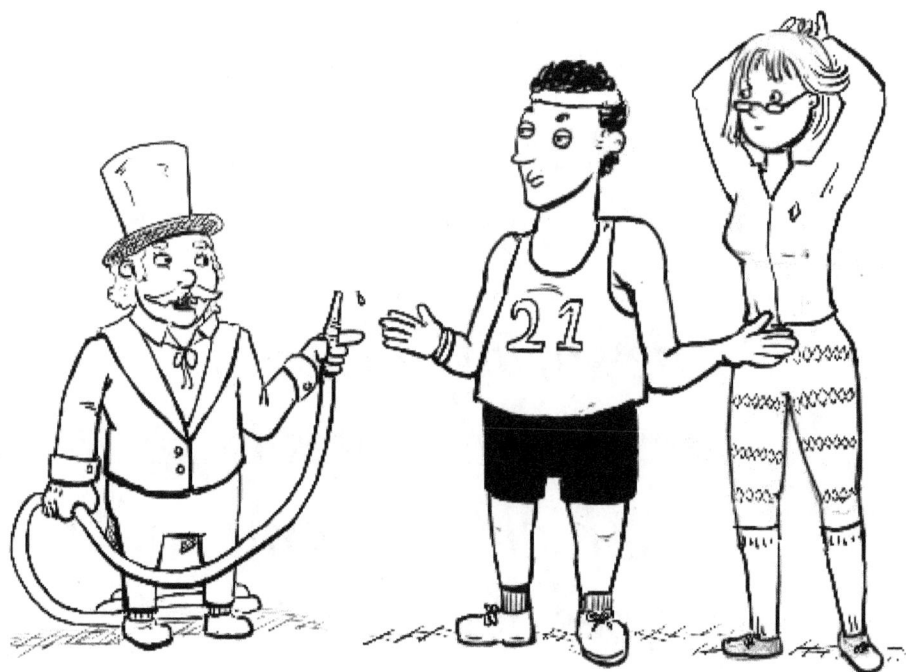

35

MYTH The Best Way to Cleanse Your Body Is Through Regular Colonics

TRUTH Colonics Have Serious Risks Such As Infection or Rectum Tear

COLONICS–ALSO CALLED COLON CLEANSES, colonic hydrotherapy or colonic irrigation–are often cited as a natural way to deal with digestive issues such as bloating, colitis, constipation and indigestion as well as other maladies not related to the gut. A colon cleanse flushes the colon with large amounts of water. For patients with constipation, it can offer immediate relief. In recent years, there have been a growing number of health claims surrounding the benefits of colonics:

- Colonics make your colon stronger
- Colonics help you lose weight
- Colonics can rid your body of harmful bacteria permanently
- Regular colon cleansing can prevent colon cancer

But here's the reality: Not a single one of these claims–none of them–is supported by any scientific research. This means the claims are not factual.

Colonics can actually be very harmful to your colon. For example, the coffee enemas currently recommended by some holistic practitioners can actually kill you, and if they don't, they can cause dehydration, increased infection risk, bowel perforation, dangerous changes in electrolytes, bloating, nausea, and vomiting. Now does that sound even the least bit healthy for your body, especially if the supposed "benefits" of colonics are not scientifically supported?

I have met with dozens of gastroenterologists in my many years of training and practice. When I ask them about colonics, they tell me this type of treatment is not a good idea and can be dangerous. The best way to make your colon happy and perform better is to watch your weight, increase the fiber and whole grains in your diet, avoid smoking, and limit alcohol. Fermented foods, greens, roughage and garlic can also be beneficial to the colon. Limiting your consumption of red meat and processed meats and avoiding too much white flour and white rice will also aid in colonic health. The single best way to protect yourself from colon cancer is a screening colonoscopy from a certified gastroenterologist.

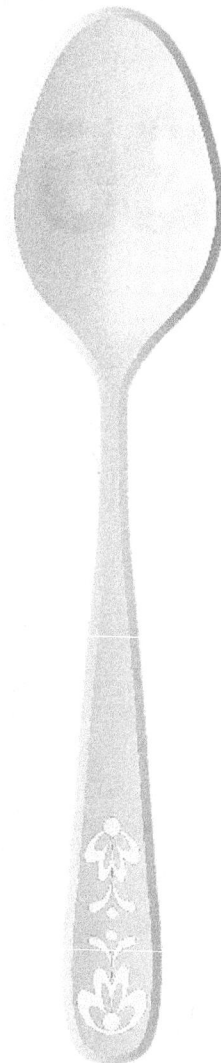

*"The single best way
to protect yourself
from colon cancer is a
screening colonoscopy
from a certified
gastroenterologist."*

"Three Parts Warm Milk, Four Parts Sleeping Pills. Sound Good?"

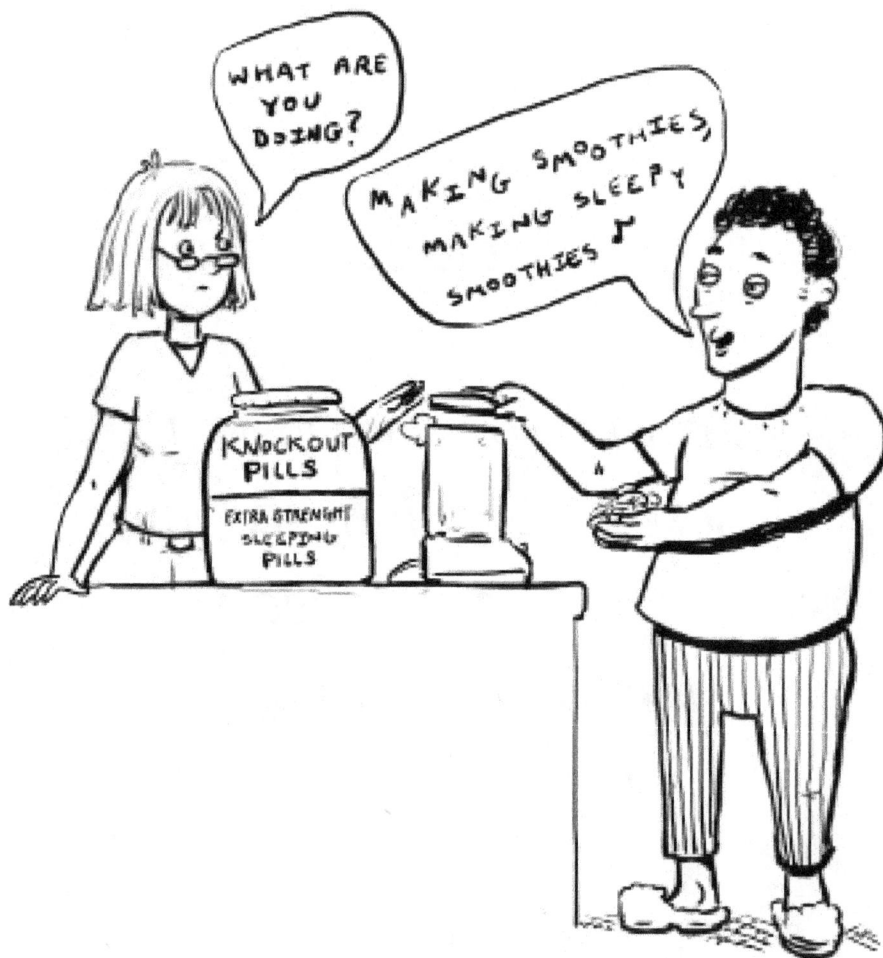

36

MYTH Prescription Sleeping Pills Aren't Dangerous

TRUTH Prescription Sleeping Pills Have Dangerous Side Effects

TAKING TOO MUCH OF SOMETHING can be dangerous, especially when it comes to medicines. Benzodiazepines (sleeping pills like Restoril®, Valium®, and Ativan®), in particular, can be habit-forming, easily misused, and are often implicated in suicides. In fact, a growing number of scientific studies associate benzodiazepines with increased mortality rates. Some recent studies also suggest that long-term use of prescription soporifics, drugs used to induce sleep, may also be implicated in the onset of dementia.

The three main classes of sleep aids are melatonin receptor agonist, benzodiazepines, and non-benzodiazepines. Melatonin has a lot of interactions with other medicines and should be carefully prescribed. Benzodiazepines are probably the riskiest sleep medicine and have potentially deadly side effects when taken with prescription painkillers. Ambien®, one of the better-known sleep aids, is a non-benzodiazepine alternative. People on Ambien® have been known to sleepwalk and may have some daytime sleepiness.

According to the National Center for Biotechnology Information, "Five studies met criteria for analysis. Low to moderate grade evidence suggests cognitive behavioral therapy for insomnia (CBT-I) has superior effectiveness to benzodiazepine and non-benzodiazepine drugs in the long term, while very low-grade evidence suggests benzodiazepines are more effective in the short term."

The biggest problem I see among my patients is that they don't prioritize sleep, so they don't get the eight hours they need. The national average in the US is about six hours of sleep a night. Some of my patients brag that they only need four hours of sleep, but seeing the bags under their eyes tells me they need more. Truth is, people who make rest a priority experience less stress in their lives and better health. If you can't sleep because of stress, learn to deal with your stress. Get the stress off your chest in the afternoon or early evening, so your mind is clear at bedtime. Also, limit media and screen time in the evening and make sure your bedroom is conducive to sleep. For example, keep the temperature a bit cooler. This can aid sleep.

If you make these changes and continue to battle with sleep issues or insomnia, don't turn to drugs. There are cognitive behavioral therapies for insomnia–including talk therapy and relaxation techniques. These techniques can help establish reliable sleep and wake patterns. Typical cognitive behavioral therapy courses last 6 to 8 weeks and are usually very effective for those struggling with sleep issues.

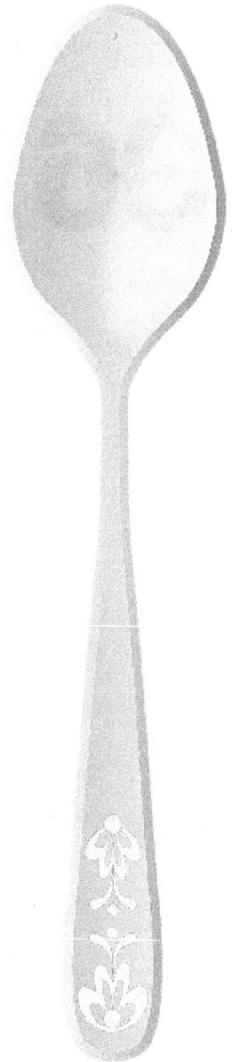

"Sleeping pills can be habit-forming."

"Just Call Me a Prescription Mixologist."

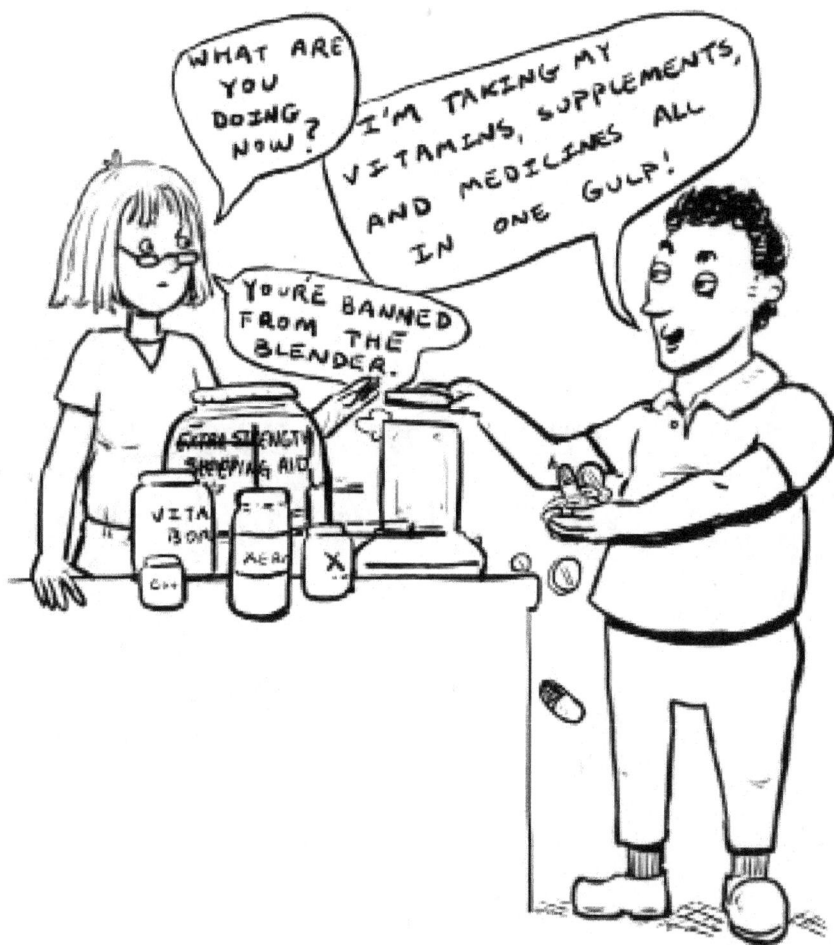

37

MYTH
Taking Over-the-counter Products Won't Interfere with Prescription Drugs

TRUTH
Over-the-counter Products Can Interfere with Prescriptions Drugs

IF YOU READ THE FINE PRINT on almost every over-the-counter drug, supplement, vitamin, or health food, you'll find a host of warnings and precautions. The human body is basically a big chemistry lab where everything from food to environmental elements to medications (both over-the-counter and prescription) interact with each other. So, let's not pretend that over-the-counter products are somehow exempt from this reality. That's not possible!

According to the Food and Drug Administration (FDA), "Drug interactions may make your drug less effective, cause unexpected side effects, or increase the action of a particular drug. Some drug interactions can even be harmful to you. Reading the label every time you use a nonprescription or prescription drug and taking the time to learn about drug interactions may be critical to your health. You can reduce the risk of potentially harmful drug interactions and side effects with a little bit of knowledge and common sense....Further, drug labels may change as new information becomes known. That's why it's especially important to read the label every time you use a drug."

Happily, these days, adverse drug interactions need never pose a quandary for anyone with a computer. There are many easy-to-use drug-interaction calculators available on the Internet. These calculators can show you interactions to look for when taking more than one medication, no matter whether over-the-counter or prescribed. Here is one of my favorites: https://healthtools.aarp.org/drug-interactions.

Do not be shy. It is important to inform your doctor about all the supplements and/or herbs you are taking as well as any other over-the-counter medications or prescription drugs. You should do this every time you see your primary care doctor. Over-the-counter aspirin, for example, may increase the risk of bleeding for those taking blood thinners like Warfarin®. Some prescription pain pills, like Norco®, contain acetaminophen. So if you take over-the-counter acetaminophen on top of that medication, you could be getting too much and doing damage to your liver.

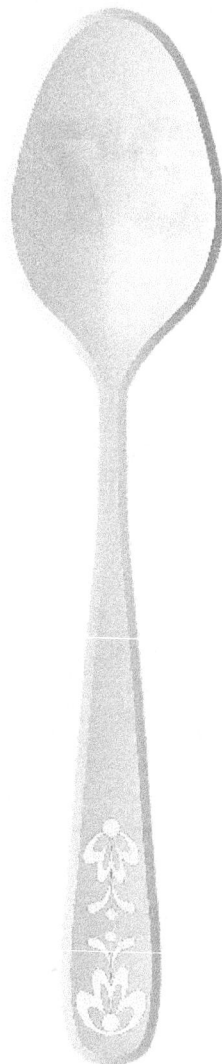

"There are many easy-to-use drug-interaction calculators available on the Internet."

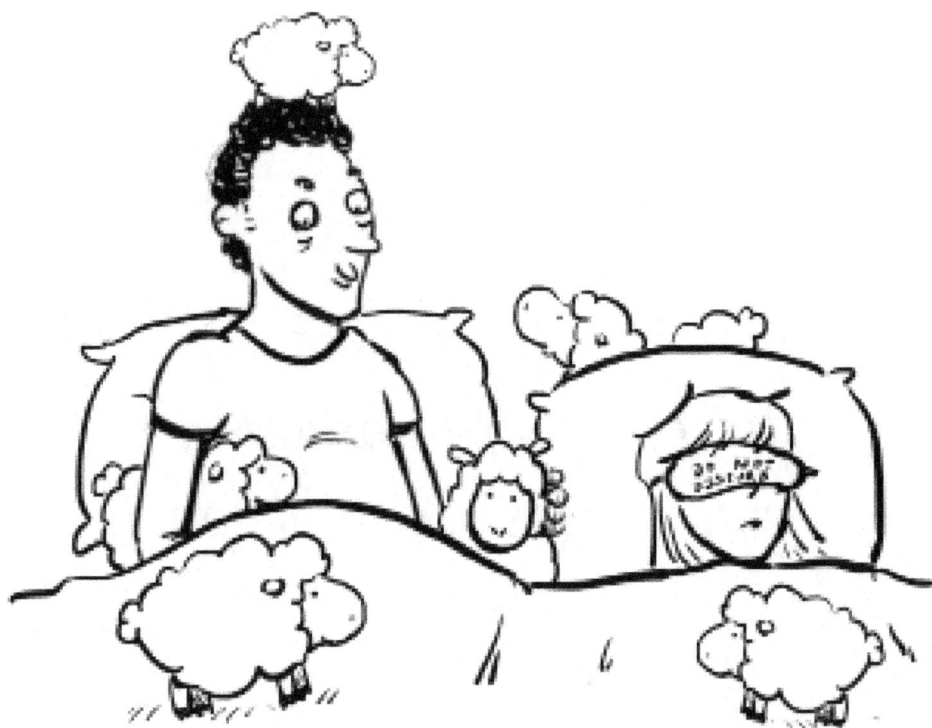

"I Need to Get Baaaaack to Sleeeep! It's Got to Work!"

38

MYTH Counting Sheep Is the Best Way To Fall Asleep

TRUTH Studies Show Counting Sheep Is Not the Best Way To Fall Asleep

SLEEP IS IMPORTANT FOR HEALTH and wellbeing. You can't live without sleep. But falling asleep and staying asleep has become a problem for many Americans. More than 60 million Americans are affected by sleep disorders every year—that's 1 in 4 Americans! And wherever there is a clustering of that many people looking for solutions, capitalism kicks in with a multitude of products and services. Sleeping pills, as discussed in an earlier myth, are one controversial solution created by the $28 billion sleep marketplace.

According to sleep.org, "One study found that people who picture a calm setting like an open field or sunset on the beach were able to fall asleep faster than those who tried to count sheep. The next time you need a quick sleep solution, consider setting aside the counting trick and imagining a waterfall, mountainside, or other pretty scene first—you could be out cold with no sheep required."

There are also Cognitive Behavioral Therapies (CBTs) that have shown positive outcomes in scientific studies about sleep. CBTs for insomnia help you identify and replace thoughts and behaviors that cause or worsen sleep problems with habits that promote sound sleep. Unlike sleeping pills, CBTs helps you overcome the underlying causes of your sleep problems.

Depending on your needs, your sleep therapist may recommend a number of CBT techniques. According to the Mayo Clinic, options include:

- **Stimulus control therapy**. This method helps remove factors that condition your mind to resist sleep. For example, you might be coached to set a consistent bedtime and wake time and avoid naps, use the bed only for sleep and sex, and leave the bedroom if you can't go to sleep within 20 minutes, only returning when you're sleepy.

- **Sleep restriction.** Lying in bed when you're awake can become a habit that leads to poor sleep. This treatment reduces the time you spend in bed, causing partial sleep deprivation, which makes you more tired the next night. Once your sleep has improved, your time in bed is gradually increased.
- **Sleep hygiene.** This method of therapy involves changing basic lifestyle habits that influence sleep, such as smoking or drinking too much caffeine late in the day, drinking too much alcohol, or not getting regular exercise. It also includes tips that help you sleep better, such as ways to wind down an hour or two before bedtime.
- **Sleep environment improvement.** This method offers ways that you can create a comfortable sleep environment, such as keeping your bedroom quiet, dark, and cool; not having a TV in the bedroom; and hiding the clock from view.
- **Relaxation training.** This method helps you calm your mind and body. Approaches include meditation, imagery, muscle relaxation and others.
- **Remaining passively awake.** Also called paradoxical intention, this involves avoiding any effort to fall asleep. Paradoxically, worrying that you can't sleep can actually keep you awake. Letting go of this worry can help you relax and make it easier to fall asleep.
- **Biofeedback.** This method allows you to observe biological signs such as heart rate and muscle tension and shows you how to adjust them. Your sleep specialist may have you take a biofeedback device home to record your daily patterns. This information can help identify patterns that affect sleep.

The most effective treatment approach may combine several of these methods. If you cannot fall asleep within about 20 minutes of going to bed, get out of bed and try some guided visualization or other relaxation techniques. I remember my mother telling me when I was a boy, rest is important, Dominic, think happy thoughts about our family vacation and you'll fall asleep. She was right. It worked!

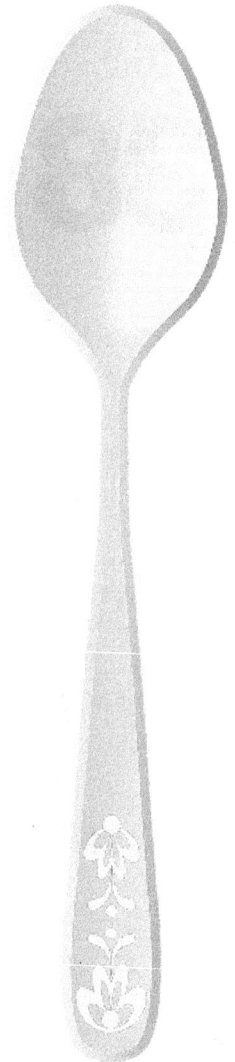

"People who pictured a calm setting like an open field or sunset on the beach were able to fall asleep faster than those who tried to count sheep."

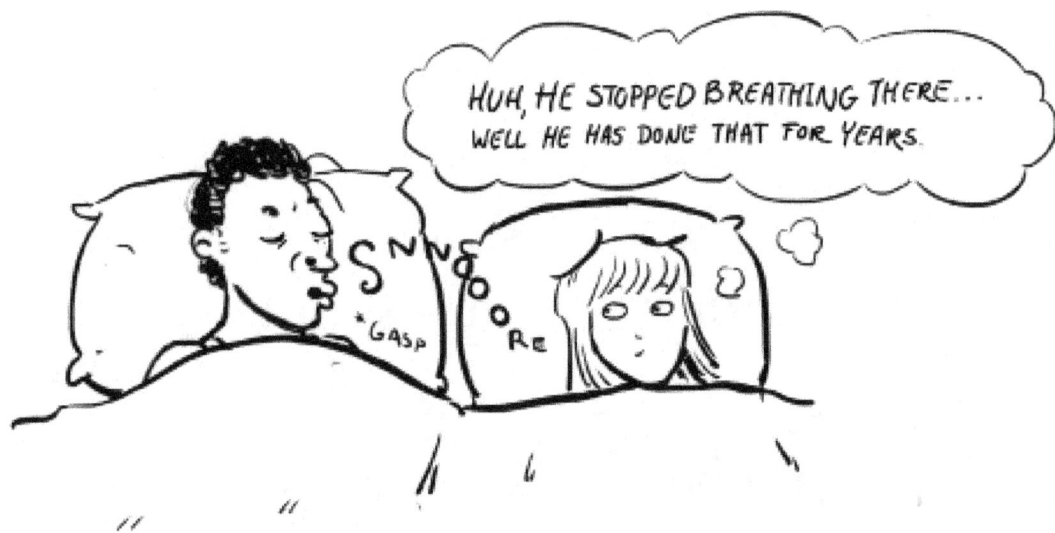

"I Need Earplugs!"

39

MYTH Snoring Is Annoying, But It's Never Dangerous

TRUTH Snoring Can Be a Sign of a Life-threatening Condition

EVERYONE SNORES, RIGHT? ACTUALLY, 45 percent of adults snore—25 percent habitually. But more than 50 million people in the United States suffer from a chronic sleep disorder that hinders their daily functioning and adversely impacts their health and longevity. Clinicians have identified more than 90 distinct sleep disorders, including excessive daytime sleepiness, difficulty initiating or maintaining sleep, and abnormal events that occur during sleep.

But don't take my word for it. The American Sleep Association says that "Snoring can be a clue to a more serious condition called obstructive sleep apnea (OSA) that often includes snoring but also has blockage of breathing during sleep. About half of patients with snoring that regularly wakes up other people will have OSA. Obstructive sleep apnea—especially severe obstructive sleep apnea—is associated with health problems like high blood pressure and increased risks of heart attack, stroke, or death."

How can you know if your snoring is a sign of a bigger sleep problem? According to the National Sleep Foundation: "People who snore make a vibrating, rattling, noisy sound while breathing during sleep. It may be a symptom of sleep apnea. Consult your doctor if you snore and have any of the following symptoms or signs:

- Excessive daytime sleepiness
- Morning headaches
- Recent weight gain
- Awakening in the morning not feeling rested
- Awaking at night feeling confused

- Change in your level of attention, concentration, or memory
- Observed pauses in breathing during sleep

If you suspect you have a problem, the definitive study for obstructive sleep apnea is an overnight sleep test that has to be done at a special facility. If a treatment is recommended, it could include one or more of the following:

- Lifestyle modification, such as sleep position training for treatment of allergies
- Surgery to address anatomical factors, like oversized tonsils
- Appliances such as nasal dilators
- Continuous Positive Airway Pressure appliance (CPAP), which blows room air into the back of the throat, thus preventing it from collapse

When I suspect sleep apnea in one of my patients, I refer them to an Ear Nose and Throat (ENT) specialist or a pulmonologist, who might order an overnight sleep study to properly diagnose their condition. Weight gain and smoking are the main contributors to the development of sleep apnea. It is important to limit alcohol consumption and be careful with certain prescription drugs like muscle relaxants, pain medication, and especially opioids. They can cause respiratory suppression, a breathing disorder characterized by slow and ineffective breathing. Sleeping on your back makes the tongue relax back further and tends to make sleep obstruction and apnea worse. If you have sleep apnea, it is recommended that you sleep on your side.

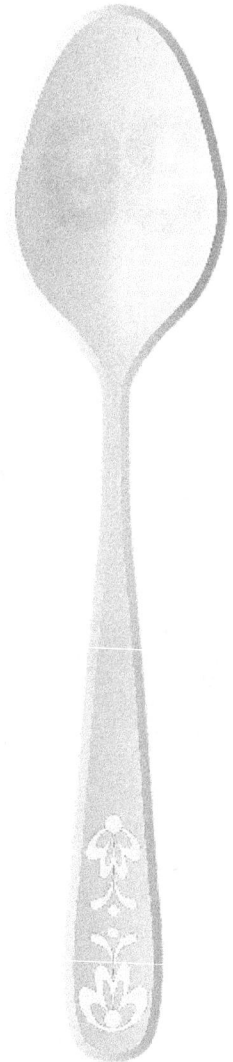

"If you suspect you have a problem, the definitive study for sleep apnea is an overnight sleep test that has to be done at a special facility."

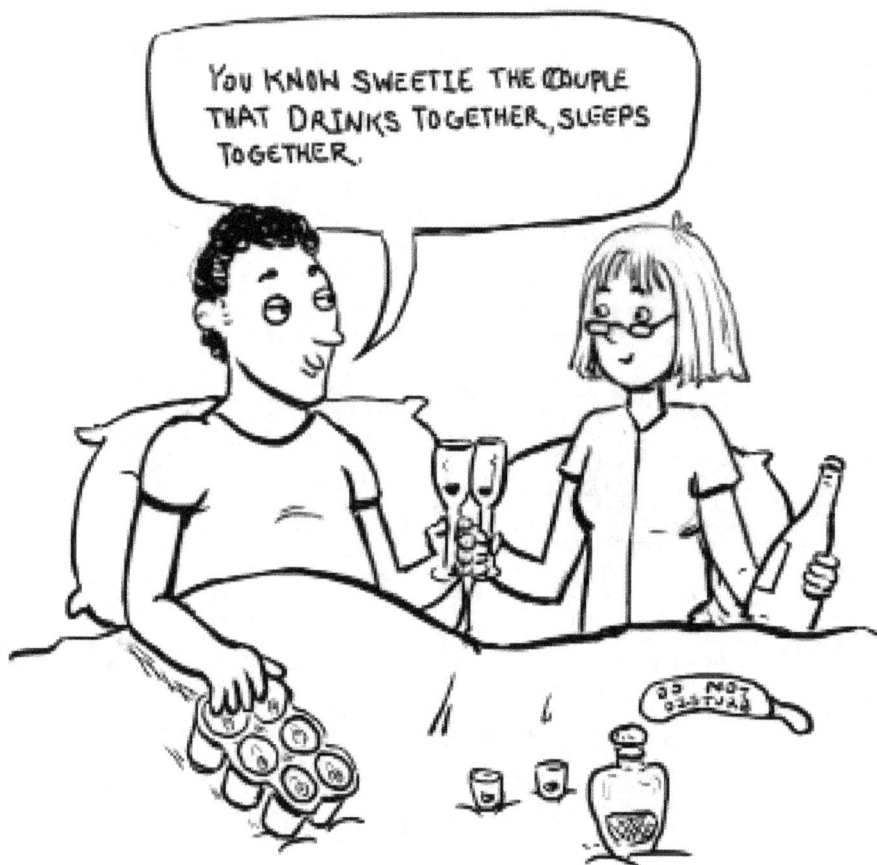

"Who Needs Sleeping Pills When You Can Have Champagne!"

40

MYTH Drinking Alcohol Leads to a Better Night's Sleep

TRUTH Alcohol Can Help You Fall Asleep, But Ruins Restorative Sleep Patterns

ALCOHOL IS A DEPRESSANT AND CAN certainly help you fall asleep. But the reality is, it contributes to poor quality sleep later in the night. More importantly, over time, alcohol use can cause lots of sleep-related problems. The National Sleep Foundation lists the following impacts of alcohol on sleep:

- Alcohol can interfere with your brain's natural sleep patterns, especially those that support the kind of deep sleep that allows for memory formation and learning.
- Alcohol increases the production of adenosine (a sleep-inducing chemical in the brain), which is why you fall asleep quickly when drinking. However, the chemical subsides as quickly as it came, making you more likely to wake up before you're truly rested.
- Alcohol blocks REM sleep, which is often considered the most restorative type of sleep. With less REM sleep, you're likely to wake up feeling groggy and unfocused.
- Alcohol causes your whole body to relax, including the muscles of your throat. And that makes you more prone to snoring and sleep apnea.
- As a diuretic, alcohol can lead to more trips to the restroom during the night, interrupting your normal sleep pattern.

My advice to those of you who have trouble falling asleep is to try something other than alcohol. Here are ten tips to fall asleep fast–and they don't have any negative side effects:

- Get on a regular schedule for going to sleep and waking up
- Lower the temperature in your bedroom
- Make sure there is no extra light in your bedroom
- Avoid high-carb foods before bed

- Turn off all electronics
- Limit caffeine intake after 3pm
- Read before bed
- Visualize things that make you happy (if sheep don't make you happy, then don't count sheep!)
- Adjust your sleep position
- Practice journaling before bed

There is a famous quote about alcohol from Shakespeare's play *Macbeth* in which the porter says, "drinking stimulates desire but hinders performance." In other words, alcohol is not a good solution. When my patients say they've turned to alcohol to help them fall asleep, I promptly redirect them to healthier, more effective alternatives.

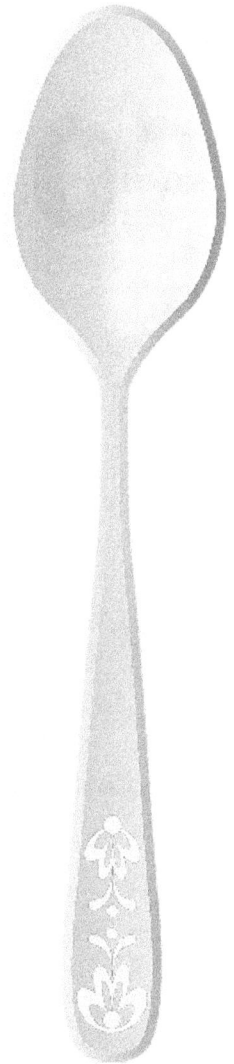

"Alcohol blocks REM sleep, which is often considered the most restorative type of sleep."

"Son, the Truth Just Doesn't Matter Sometimes."

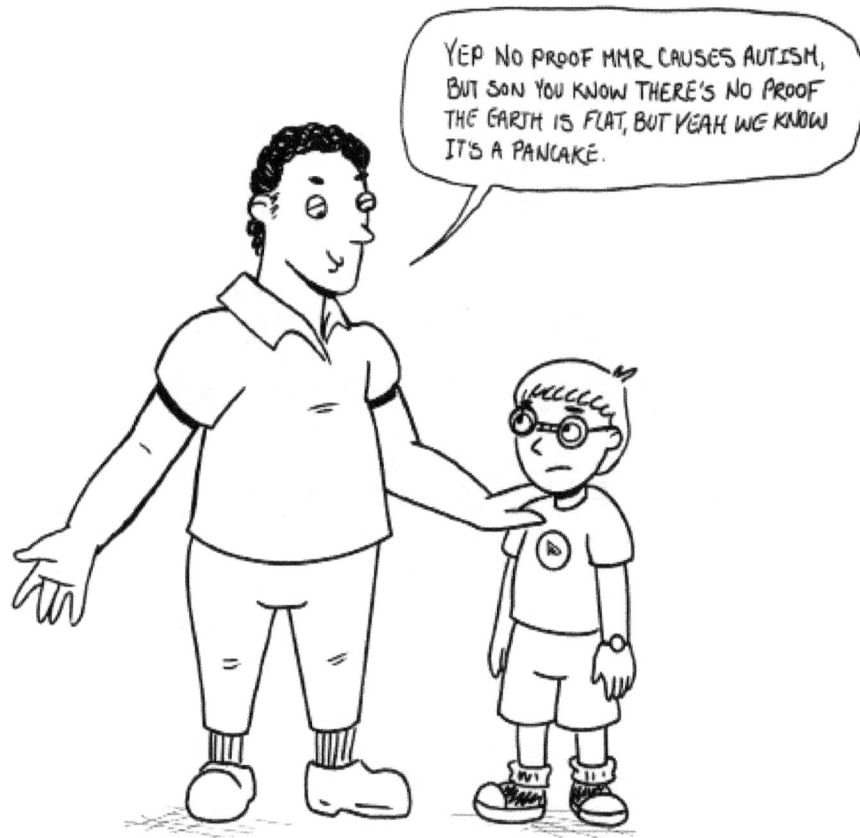

MYTH 41

MYTH The Mumps, Measles, Rubella Vaccine (MMR) Causes Autism

TRUTH There Is Absolutely No Evidence That an MMR Causes Autism

The idea that the Measle, Mumps, Rubella (MMR) vaccine causes autism started back in 1998, when the British medical journal, *The Lancet,* published a paper by Dr. Andrew Wakefield that claimed to document a clear connection between the two. The fraudulent paper was ultimately retracted by *The Lancet,* its science totally repudiated, and its author stripped of his medical license after "Britain's General Medical Council ruled that the children that Wakefield studied were carefully selected and some of Wakefield's research was funded by lawyers acting for parents who were involved in lawsuits against vaccine manufacturers."

Unfortunately, the retraction didn't do the trick. It was too late to put the genie back in the bottle. The idea that the MMR vaccine caused autism stuck and spread across the globe. It is perhaps the most widely accepted medical myth of our time. Unfortunately, its acceptance has created a dangerous movement in which parents opt out of some or all immunizations for their children. "Vaccine hesitancy" is now a major movement in the United States. In some areas of the country, vaccination coverage is slipping below the 90 to 95 percent coverage rate that experts say is needed to prevent outbreaks.

Dozens of studies explored the possible connection between vaccination and autism and no connection of any kind has ever been found—not one...ever. Luckily, the vast majority of Americans know that vaccinations save lives and prevent illness. They participate in a regular immunization schedule. But recent outbreaks of measles in areas of the United States where vaccine hesitancy has taken hold point to our need to continually monitor and educate.

Some 15 million children have been studied since 1998 and no link has been shown between the MMR and autism. If others would look at these studies, as I did, they would see the clear reasons why no association between the MMR vaccine and autism exists. But once people believe medical misinformation, it's difficult to convince them otherwise. One of my favorite YouTube channels, which I show my medical students, was created by a passionate pediatrician named Dr. Aaron Carroll. His "Healthcare Triage" channel has a lot of great videos. As a pediatrician, he cares deeply about children and autism. In episode 12 of "Healthcare Triage," Dr. Carroll brings together the research findings in "Vaccines Don't Cause Autism." His advice: We should focus on the best ways to help autistic children flourish and fund more basic scientific research where it can really make a difference.

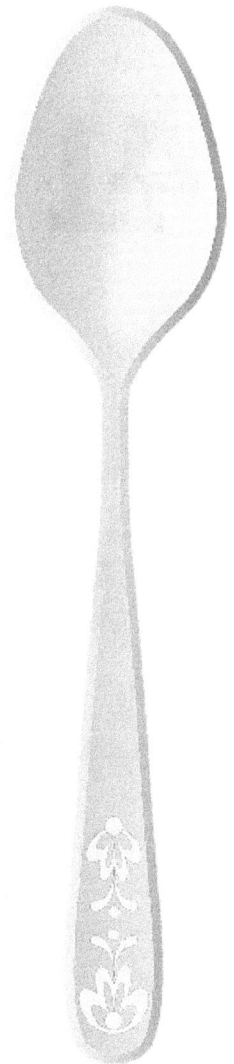

"15 million children have been studied since 1998 and no link has been shown between the MMR and autism.

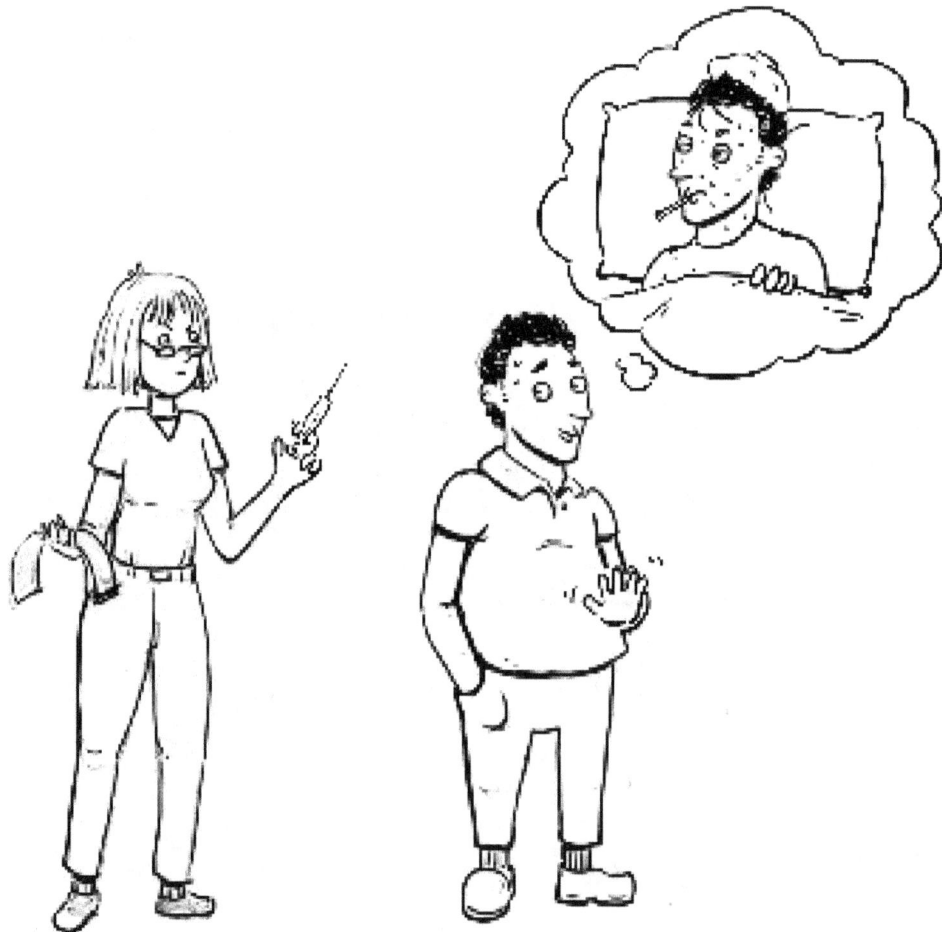

"I'm Not Taking That Vaccine. No Way!"

42 MYTH The Flu Vaccine Causes the Flu

TRUTH It's Not Possible for the Flu Shot To Give You the Flu

THE IDEA THAT THE FLU SHOT can cause the flu is a very popular myth among all my patients. When I ask some of my patients if they would like a flu shot, they wave me off confidently. "No, doctor, absolutely not," they tell me. Since I believe the flu shot is important, I stop to ask them why they choose not to take this precaution before flu season. I always take the time to address their concerns.

It is impossible to get the flu from the flu vaccine because the virus has been inactivated. Therefore, it is not infectious. If you think skipping the flu shot is less risky than getting the vaccine, you are wrong. Approximately 60,000 people in America die each year from flu complications. Yes, these victims are primarily the very young, the elderly, and those with chronic medical conditions. However, in recent years, doctors have seen an increased number of healthy, middle-age adults suffer and die from various complications like a viral myocarditis or heart infection. The bottom line is that the flu is not a benign disease, and the absolute best way to protect you, your family, and your whole community from the flu is to get vaccinated.

Over the years, a handful of patients have come to me after receiving the flu vaccine and believed they have suffered a side effect from the shot. After discussing their symptoms, I have been able to reassure them that their symptoms were not a side effect of the flu shot. In fact, I have never seen any of my patients suffer a side effect from the flu vaccine. As a result of my proactive approach to patient education about the flu shot, I'm happy to report that more than 90 percent of my patient population receives the vaccine during flu season, year after year.

On my honor, you will not catch the flu from the vaccine. It's not a possibility, so say goodbye to that myth and say hello to the immunity boost your system needs before flu season hits.

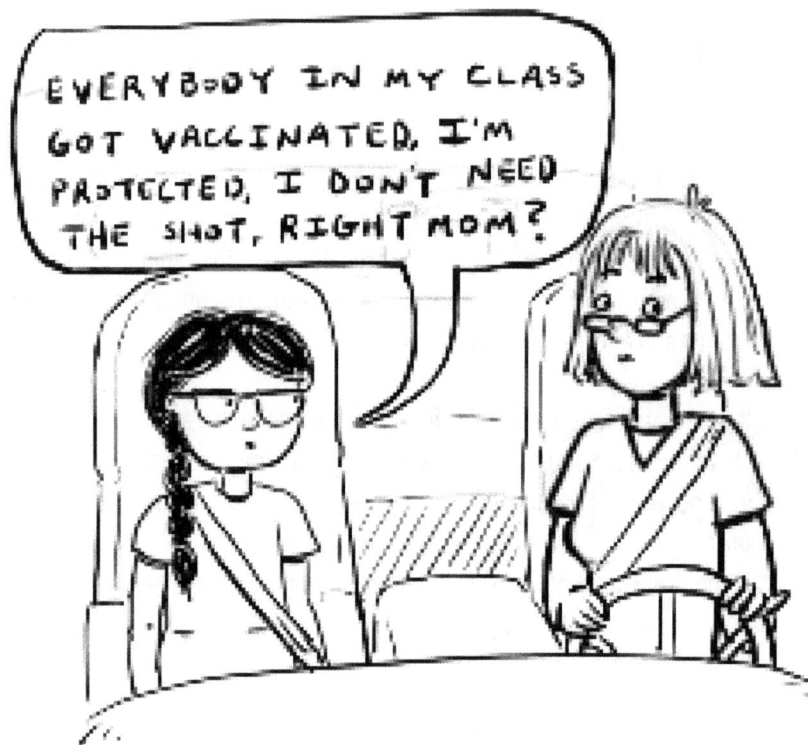

"Should I Be a Good Mom or a Cool Mom?"

43

MYTH My Child Doesn't Need Vaccines Because Other Kids Are Vaccinated

TRUTH Vaccine Programs Rely on High Levels of Participation To Be Effective

TO UNDERSTAND WHY YOUR CHILD needs to be vaccinated even if others around your child have already been immunized, you need to understand the concept of "herd immunity." If everybody in your family and community has been administered a flu shot, then everybody in that group is protected. If 7 out of 10 in your group gets the flu shot, then you are most likely all protected. But if only 4 out of the 10 gets the flu shot, it becomes more likely that unimmunized people in the group will get the flu. There's a threshold in immunization coverage that has to be met to tip the scales and protect a population. So please do your part to educate your family and friends about the importance of vaccinations.

The Centers for Disease Control and Prevention, shares these 6 things you should know about vaccines

- We all need vaccines throughout our lives to help protect against serious diseases.
- Outbreaks of vaccine-preventable diseases can, and do, still happen in communities across the US
- The CDC and FDA take many steps to make sure vaccines are very safe.
- Vaccines give you the power to protect your children from getting sick.
- You can even make sure your baby is born with protection by getting vaccinated when you are pregnant.
- Vaccines aren't just for kids. They can help adults stay healthy too–especially if they have health conditions.

Getting you and your child vaccinated when indicated by your health care provider is essential to provide immunity before exposure to potentially life-threatening diseases.

Vaccines are rigorously tested before they are administered to the public to ensure that they are safe and effective for children to receive at the recommended age.

The World Health Organization (WHO) has declared vaccine hesitancy as a top-10 problem in the world, as the number of cases of measles has tripled in Europe and are the highest in years in the United States. The main reason for these outbreaks is a break in "herd immunity" in various countries across the world. Immunization numbers are falling, and this puts everyone in danger. To protect against measles in the United States, many experts say we need 95 percent of the country vaccinated against measles, which is a very contagious and dangerous virus.

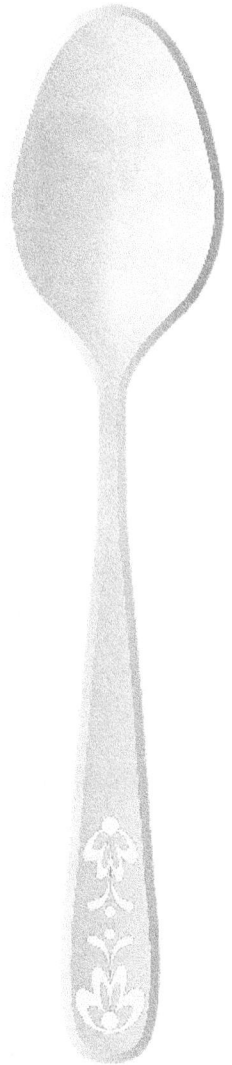

"The World Health Organization has declared vaccine hesitancy as a top-10 problem in the world."

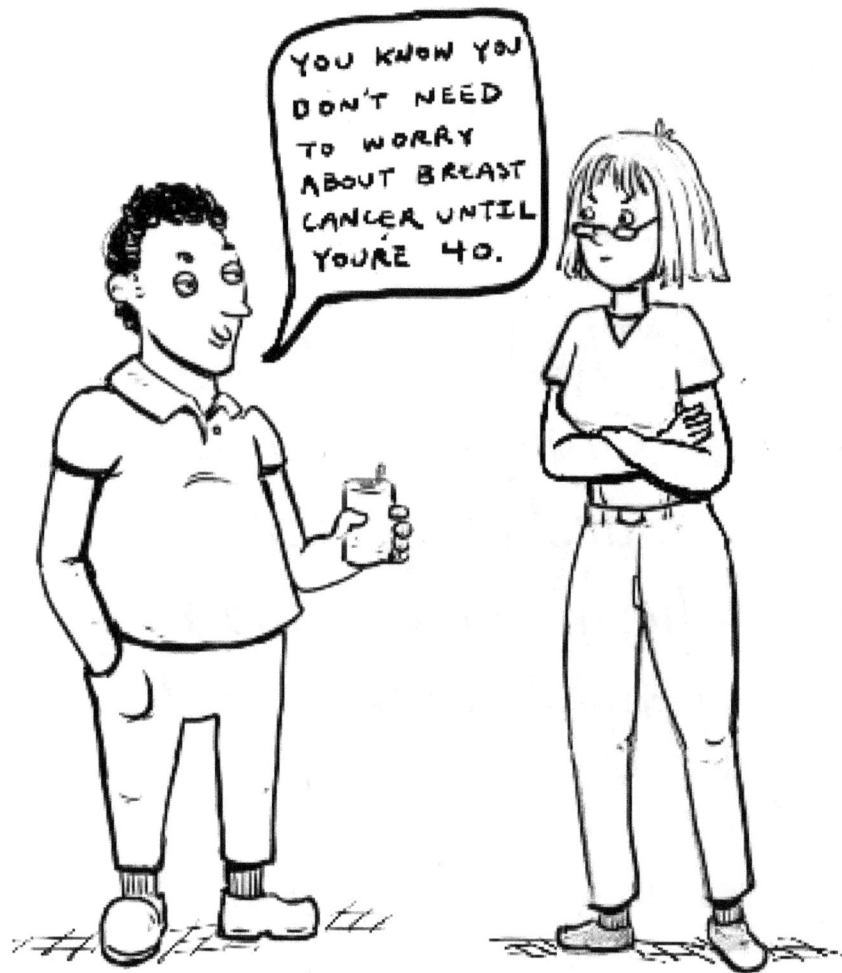
"Did He Just Tell Me What To Do With My Body?"

MYTH 44

MYTH Mammograms Aren't Benificial for Women Under the Age of 50

TRUTH Mammograms Can Be Benificial for Women Under the Age of 50, Especially Those at Higher Risk

HERE ARE THE SCREENING GUIDELINES: The US Preventive Services Task Force modified its screening recommendations for mammograms to begin at age 50, and the American Cancer Society (ACS) recommends women begin screening at age 45. This might be fine for women who don't have any of the known risk factors for breast cancer, but it's not good advice for women who do. Okay, so this is sort of a "caveat myth," but the caveat is *very* important, in fact it could save a life.

I selected this as a myth because it's too easy for women to listen to the popular age recommendations for a mammogram without knowing whether they have any risk factors in their medical history. If you have any of the risk factors listed below (particularly the first one), then you should consider getting a baseline mammogram when you're as young as 30. Then, you should make an annual mammography part of your health-maintenance routine. Here are the risk factors:

- A family history of breast cancer, particularly in direct female relatives (for example, your mother)
- A personal history of breast cancer
- A biopsy showing malignant markers
- Any history of radiation therapy
- Clinical finding of BRCA1/BRCA2 gene mutation

If you don't have any of the risk factors on this list, then you can probably safely wait for a mammography until you turn 50, when your longevity-related risks for the disease increase.

157

According to the ACS, "There is no sure way to prevent breast cancer. But there are things you can do that might lower your risk. This can be especially helpful for women with certain risk factors for breast cancer, such as having a strong family history or certain gene changes." The organization makes these suggestions:

- Stay at a healthy weight and get regular exercise
- Limit your alcohol intake
- Eat a diet that is rich in vegetables, fruit, poultry, fish, and low-fat dairy products

For women at increased risk of breast cancer–due to a strong family history with the disease, for example–there are prescription medications that can be used to help lower the risk for some women. This risk is assessed using something called the Gail Model. If a woman's breast cancer risk is determined to be high, "Prescription medicines can be used to help lower breast cancer risk in certain women at increased risk of breast cancer," the ACS writes. "...Medicines such as tamoxifen and raloxifene block the action of estrogen in breast tissue. Tamoxifen can be taken even if you haven't gone through menopause, while raloxifene is only used for women who have gone through menopause. Other drugs, called *aromatase inhibitors*, might also be an option for women past menopause. All of these medicines can have side effects, so it's important to understand the possible benefits and risks of taking them.

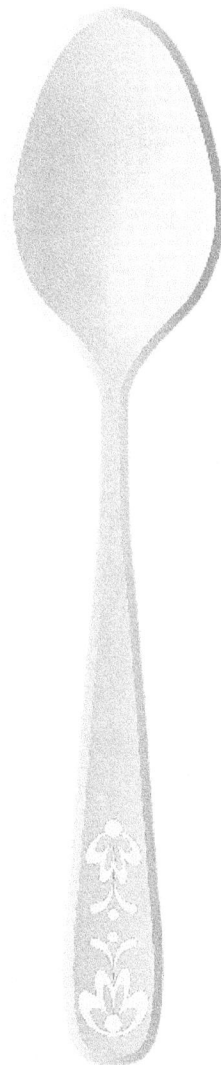

"There are prescription medications that can be used to help lower the breast cancer risk for some women."

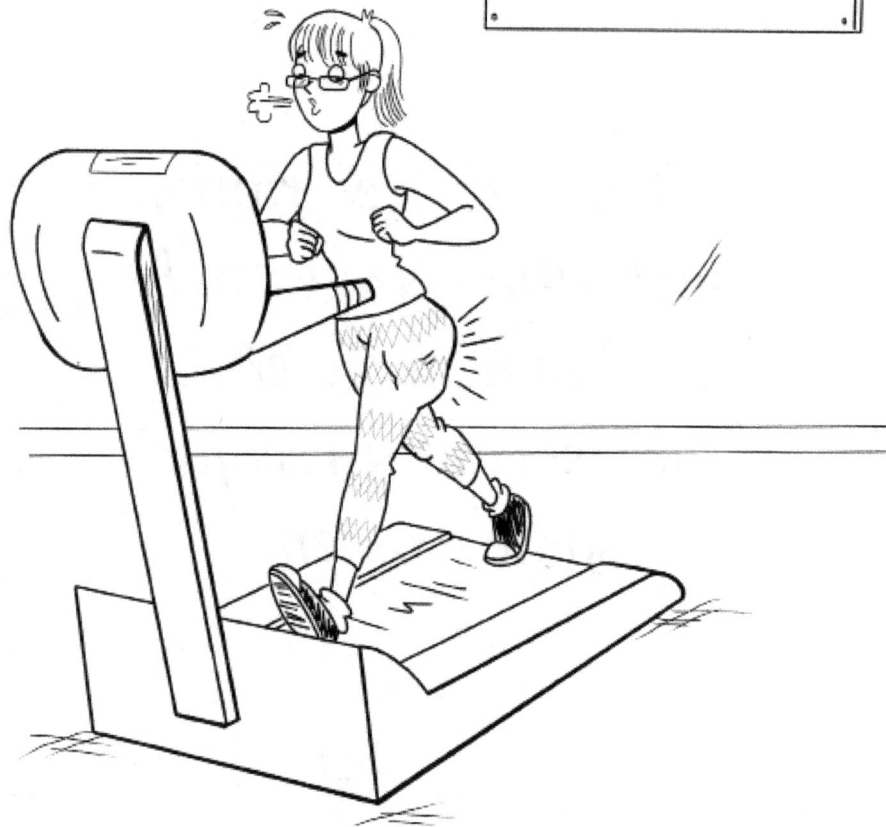

"I Wonder If Focus, Focus Is Really Hocus Pocus!"

LEFT HIP BURNER

45

MYTH Machines and Certain Exercises Can Target Weight Loss Toward Specific Body Parts

TRUTH These "Target" Tactics Do Not Lead to Fat Reduction in That Area

FIRST OF ALL, I wonder why certain people gain fat in one particular area of the body. The fat deposition is based on your sex, age, lifestyle and genetics. Women have a higher percentage of body fat than men and tend to have excess fat in the thighs and buttocks, especially during childbearing years. Men are more likely to put on weight in their abdomen.

Spot reduction is the effort to remove a particular area of fat by exercising the associated muscle. Studies have shown that exercising one particular muscle group will certainly show gains in muscle and look better cosmetically in that area because of the muscle shaping. However, it does not specifically reduce fat in those areas.

Many of my patients are concerned about how they look and why they have developed fat in certain areas. Most of the time, it is related to their sex, genetics or some other contributing factor. For example, some patients come to me with enlarged legs and think they are swollen. When I examine them, I do not see any fluid, only a deposit of fatty tissue in their legs. Fat deposits can also be a side effect of medical syndromes called Cushing Syndrome, in which an excess of hormones leads the patient to develop a rounded face and fat deposits in the upper back. This is often called a buffalo hump. A similar fat deposit can occur when my patients are on long-term steroids.

The bottom line is that there is no real scientific evidence that you can lose weight in a particular part of the body by exercising that part of the body.

"The Pap Smear Blues."

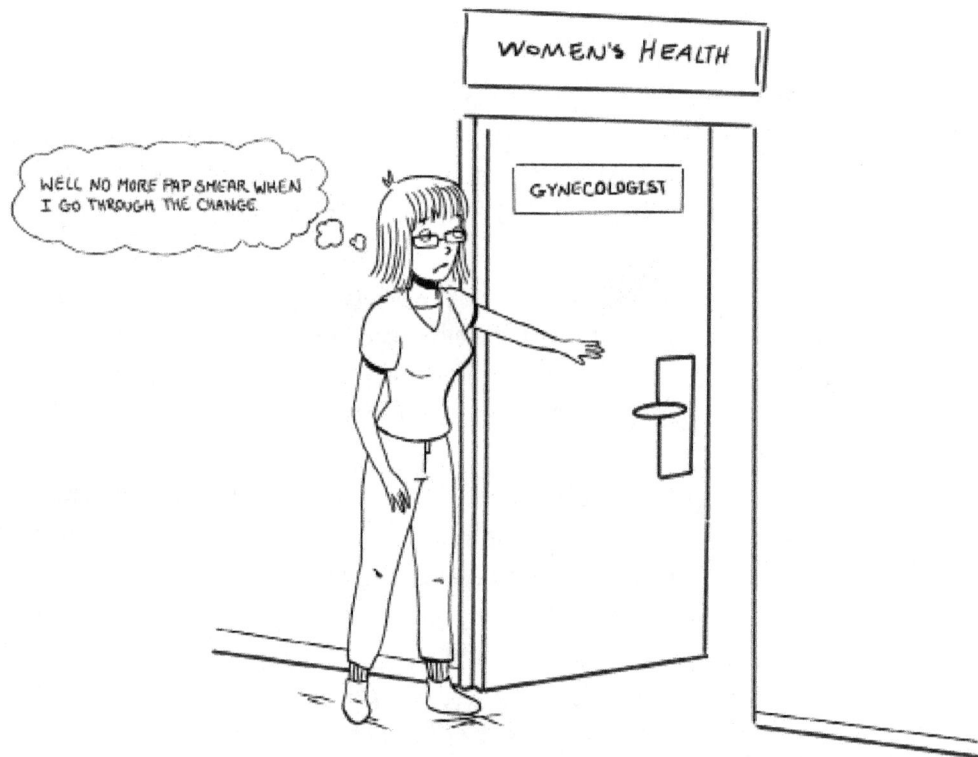

46

MYTH You Don't Need a Pap Smear After Menopause

TRUTH Pap Smears Are an Important Test for Adult Women up to Age 65

According to the US task force on screenings, a PAP smear is a Level-A screening test, meaning it offers the highest category of screening to detect disease. But most post-menopausal women believe they can safely stop routine PAP smear testing once they are through menopause. But that's not what the US Preventative Service Task Force (USPSTF) recommends.

Remember, the risk of almost all cancers increases with age. If you still have a cervix, you still face some risk of contracting cervical cancer. And while having a hysterectomy prevents uterine cancer, if your uterus was removed because of a cancerous or precancerous condition, then your risk of cervical cancer is elevated. So, if you have had any of the known risk factors for cervical cancer, you should continue regular Pap testing until your doctor suggests it is safe to stop. The most important risk factor for cervical cancer is infection with the Human Papilloma Virus (HPV), commonly known as the Herpes virus. Other risk factors are:

- Positive HIV/AIDS test
- Immune system deficiency
- History of smoking
- Use of oral contraceptives

Cervical cancer is one of those diseases that, if caught early, it is very treatable. But about 20 percent of the diagnoses are for women over 65 years of age. Pap smears aren't fun, but there are absolutely no known risks or side effects of a Pap smear screening, so what is the downside? The upside is that you could catch a problem early and save your life. That's a pretty big upside, if you ask me.

163

The five-year survival rate for early stage cervical cancer is about 90 percent. USPSTF recommends screening for cervical cancer for women 21 to 65 years old, with cytology every three years. Those women that want to lengthen the screening interval from age 30 to 65 can do so with a combination of cytology and HPV testing every five years.

Many of my patients do not want to do screening because they are afraid of what they might find. But it is important to know the truth, so you have a variety of treatment options. A patient's treatment options often narrow as the disease progresses. Turn to friends, family and your primary care doctor for support in dealing with a difficult diagnosis. If you have an abnormal Pap smear, it is advised to have a separate visit to go over your results, if you have an abnormal Pap smear. The Pap smear is very effective for detecting cervical cancer, so don't avoid getting the test just because it is uncomfortable. Most of the time, the results are actually good news and will relieve your anxiety.

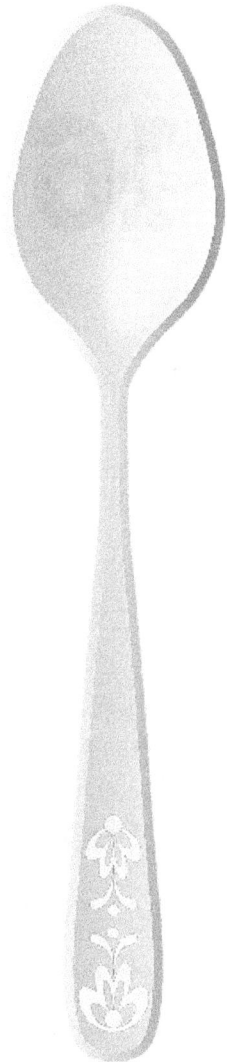

"If you still have a cervix, you still face some risk of contracting cervical cancer."

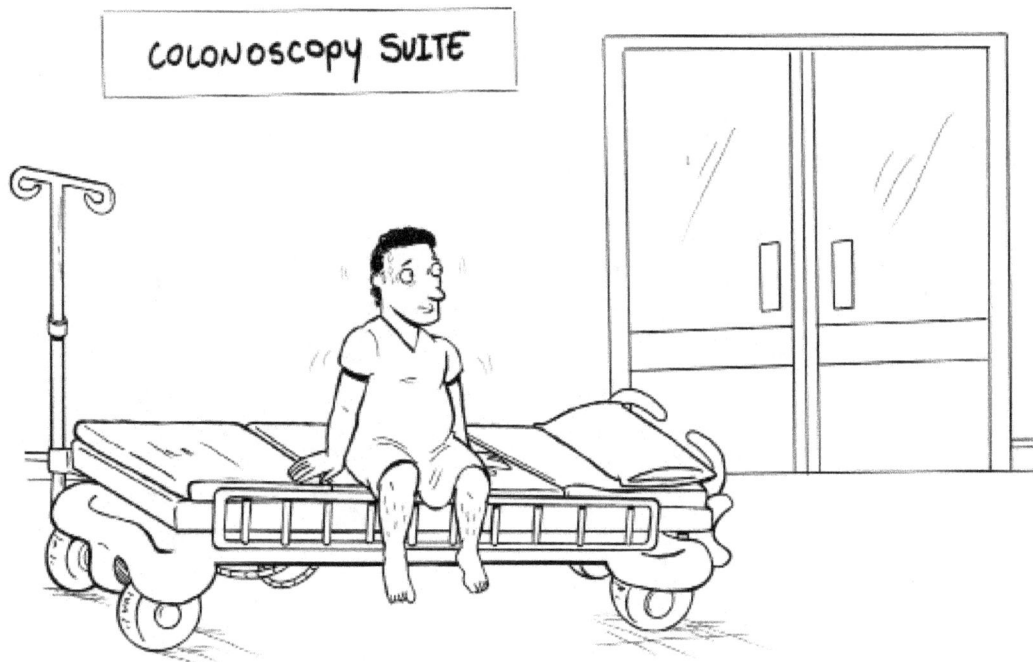

47

MYTH Colonoscopies Are Very Painful

TRUTH Colonoscopies Are Uncomfortable, But Very Important

COLONOSCOPIES ARE THE SINGLE BEST DEFENSE against colon and rectal cancer–also referred to as colorectal cancer–is the fourth most common type of cancer in the US. An estimated 135,000 new cases of colorectal cancer are diagnosed each year and it causes roughly 50,000 deaths.

Even if colonoscopies were painful, I would continue to recommend them to my patients as they turn 50 years old, which is the recommended age to establish a baseline for your colon health. Believe me, I understand that the thought of a tube going up you colon is unsettling. Yest, it *is* an uncomfortable procedure. But the benefits of a colonoscopy far outweigh the discomfort. Even if you are highly sensitive, there are solutions. Read on...

In addition to diagnostic benefits, colonoscopies can also prevent cancer. How? "Colon cancer universally starts off as a polyp that's been allowed to grow and to generate into a cancer," said Dr. Lina O'Brien, who regularly performs colonoscopies. "So, if you can remove the polyp before it has a chance to change, you can eliminate the cancer from forming."

A polyp is a small growth that forms in the lining of the colon. When you have a colonoscopy, the surgeon is inspecting the entire colon, the rectum and part of the small bowel. If the doctors find a polyp along the way, they remove it. If it is too big to remove, they can biopsy it. Since even benign polyps can turn into cancer later, any polyp too large to be removed during the colonoscopy will require surgery (at a later date).

I've had many patients who regularly undergo their colonoscopies with no anesthetic or sedative at all. But for those who are highly sensitive to pain, doctors who perform colonoscopies have a whole arsenal of sedatives and anesthetics available to make the procedure totally pain-free—as in you won't feel a thing. Most patients ask me whether the gastroenterologist performing the colonoscopy will put them to sleep. This type of anesthetic is up to the discretion of the gastroenterologist. Most of the time, though, sedatives are sufficient.

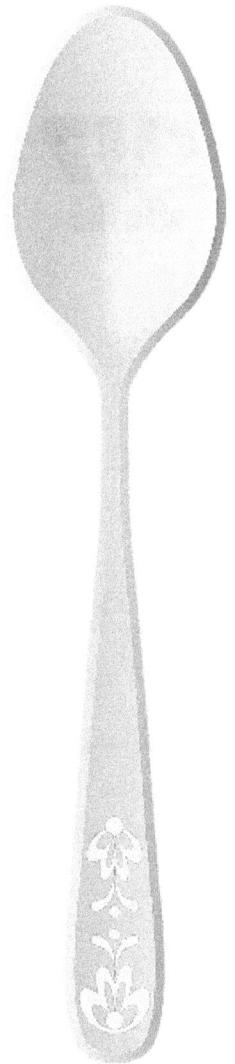

"The benefits of a colonoscopy far outweigh the discomfort."

"I Don't Think It Works That Way."

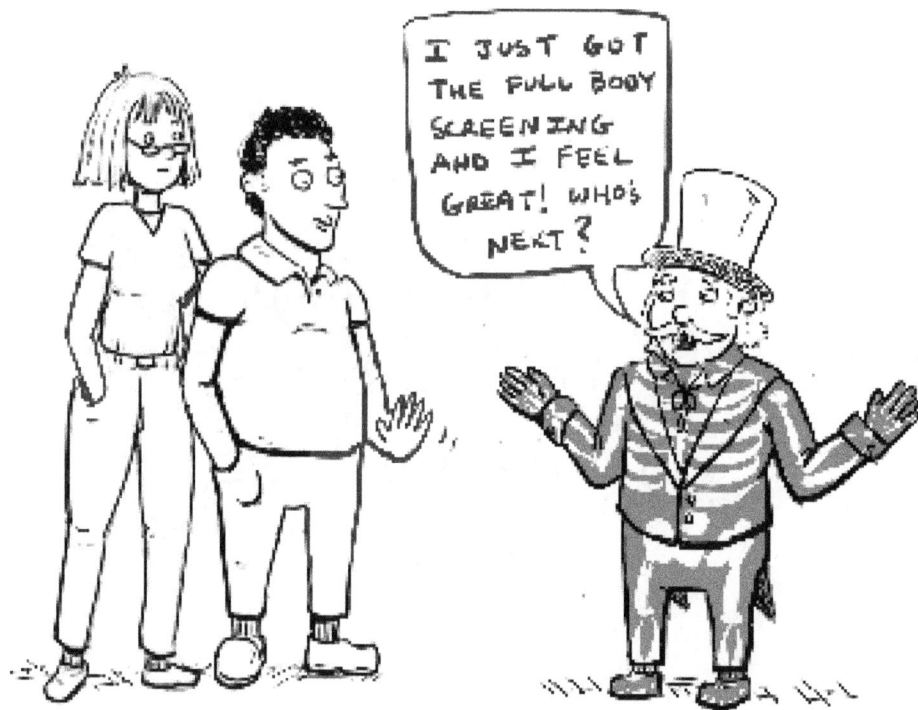

48

MYTH Whole-body Screening Is a Good Way to Detect Hidden Cancers

TRUTH Whole-body Screening Is Not a Reliable Screening Tool for Cancer

When my patients come in to be screened for cancer, they often ask if there is one specific test that I can give them to rule out all cancers. Unfortunately, it doesn't work that way. Some of my patients have heard about whole-body screening and think that's the test that will reveal if they have cancer. Whole-body screening is often a very useful follow-up tool for tracking a patient's progress after he or she has had cancer treatment, especially if the initial tumor is known to be metastatic. But when it comes to routine whole-body screenings, which have become big business in the US and Canada, the experts have said it best:

"There is no evidence that whole-body screening of healthy people prevents cancer-related deaths. In fact, evidence shows that whole-body screening—which is neither sensitive nor specific—poses a number of serious risks to patients....Whole-body screening also increases the rate of over-diagnosis—the diagnosis of diseases or ailments that would not have caused any problems in a person's lifetime or for which therapy is not known to be effective."

As a doctor, my focus is not on some "miraculous" test that, as it turns out, isn't the solution which we'd all hoped it would be. Unfortunately, there is no single, whole-body screening test for cancer. There are many different types of cancer, so one test couldn't possibly detect all cancers. For me, the focus is on finding out about my patients' risk factors, which I have seen play a role in cancer over and over again. I want to know about a patient's lifestyle, their family history, their exposure to chemicals in the workplace, and such. I want to learn if they have any unusual symptoms. Have they lost a lot of weight lately without dieting? Are they fatigued all the time, even after a good night's rest? I also want to talk to them about what they could be doing to prevent cancer. Isn't prevention, after all, the most important goal?

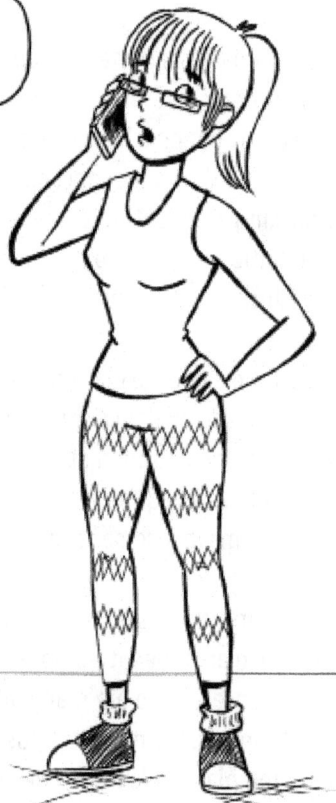

"If Jane Fonda Could Do It Every Day, Why Can't I?"

MYTH

49

MYTH To Keep Fit, You Must Work Out Hard Every Day

TRUTH Exercise Is Important, But Daily Exercise Is Not Mandatory for Health

The American Heart Association recommends moderate cardio exercise in five, 30-minute sessions a week or 35- to 40-minute sessions a few times each week. And, if your workouts are more vigorous, there's a bonus: you only need 75 minutes of exercise a week or three, 25-minute sessions. Anything that gets your heart rate up–running, dancing, swimming, cycling or rowing–counts as a cardio workout.

The interesting thing is the American Heart Association hasn't established a guideline for what constitutes too much exercise. Researchers are just starting to look at this side of exercise, and they've made some interesting observations. A paper published in The Lancet Psychiatry about the association between physical exercise and mental health found that "In a large US sample, physical exercise was significantly and meaningfully associated with self-reported mental health burden in the past month. More exercise was not always better." The researchers found that the participants who benefited most in terms of mental health were those who exercised for 30–60 minutes three to five times per week.

In a recent *US News and World Report* story entitled, "How Much Exercise is Too Much?" the contributing writer looked at a number of studies that might serve as a wake-up call for extreme athletes and those who tend to over-train. "Chronic training for and competing in extreme events...may cause short-term negative cardiovascular effects. For example, among a group of patients diagnosed with coronary artery disease, those who exercised beyond the recommended 60-minute maximum saw decreases in their antioxidant levels as well as stiffening of their blood vessels. In comparison, those exercisers who exerted themselves within a more reasonable range–i.e., in 60 minutes or less–saw a reduction in free radicals, in addition to improved circulation."

Even those who work out in a more normal range might benefit from an exercise break. As the fitness site verywellfit.com says, "It isn't bad to work out every day. Doing some form of physical activity each day is smart when you're trying to slim down. But if you want to lose weight, repeating the same workout mode, intensity, or duration day after day won't work. Why? Your body adjusts to the daily workload and you hit the dreaded weight-loss plateau."

Note to those of you who consider yourselves happy "couch potatoes" and think that I'm saying it's okay to slouch off. No way! Moderate exercise as part of your weekly routine is very beneficial for your health. Please get up off the couch and get moving! You will improve your cardiovascular health. Exercise is also a recognized treatment for anxiety and depression. Exercise helps keep blood sugar and cholesterol levels in line as well as control blood pressure. Exercise is important.

What I'm advocating is balance and moderation. In many communities, the pendulum has swung too far in the other direction. Over time, extreme endurance exercises like ultra-marathons may lead to heart damage, heart-rhythm disorders, and enlarged arteries in some people. Moderate exercise can improve your immune system, but excessive exercise can actually decrease it. Did you know that you are more likely to get a cold or bronchitis in the 72-hour "open window" of impaired immunity after intense exercise? The key to optimal life is balance.

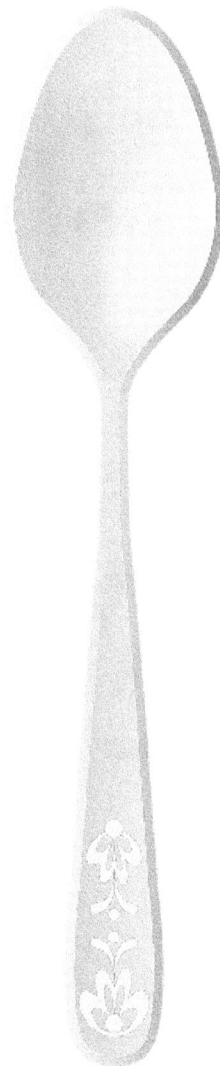

"Researchers found that participants who benefited the most in terms of mental health were those who exercised for 30-60 minutes three to five times per week."

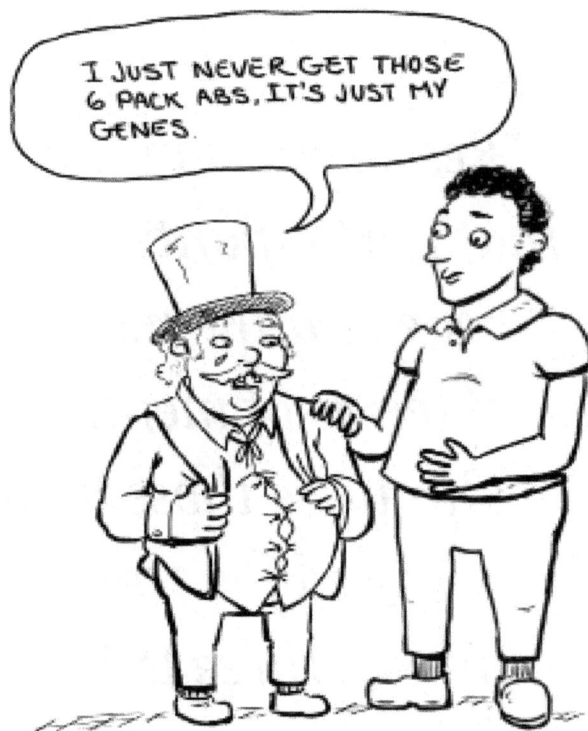

"Yep, I've Got the Fat Gene!"

50

MYTH Obesity Can't Be Reversed Because It's Genetic

TRUTH With Regard to Weight, Your Genes Are Not Your Destiny

Yes, genes play a powerful role in many aspects of our lives, but so do our lifestyle and health choices. More and more, science is finding that environmental and lifestyle choices can "trigger" genes. It might explain why some people have gene markers for specific diseases, such as breast cancer, but never actually suffer from the disease. No, your genes are not your destiny–even when it comes to your weight. According to experts at the Harvard School of Public Health:

> "The genetic factors identified so far make only a small contribution to obesity risk. Many [of the] people who carry these so-called 'obesity genes' do not become over-weight, and (in many cases) healthy lifestyles can almost completely counteract these genetic effects."

When someone comes to talk to me about their struggles with his or her weight, I start with a series of questions and a specific set of lab tests for such things as a thyroid disorder. The first thing I do is determine the patient's ideal weight. When we talk about weight, many patients are surprised by what they should weigh. I tell them ideal weight is important because this is the weight at which they are least likely to develop diabetes, high blood pressure or other diseases. An ideal weight, according to height, age and other factors, is the weight that will place the least burden on joints, bones and organs. When we decide target a weight that is ideal and to reach that weight in a reasonable amount of time, I call this the target weight and target date. A few months later, I follow up and ask my patients if they have experienced successful weight loss or not. If they were not successful, I recommend that they keep a food and exercise diary for the next three weeks and come back and see me. Often times, my patients are not aware of their daily food and exercise choices.

When they write them down, they start to see patterns. The become more accountable to themselves. It's a valuable tool, if you're trying to change habits.

Dr. Eddie Fatakhov, a board-certified internist and nutritionist, told healthline.com that there is hope for people who are battling their weight, even if they have the so called "obesity gene." He says, "Take it one day at a time. Sustainable weight loss is a marathon, not a sprint. It does nobody any good to lose 30 pounds, then gain it back 6 months later." He suggests working with medical experts and keeping a food journal. I agree with both of these strategies.

There are amazing digital controls that you can use on your computer or smartphone, the best I know is the highly rated "Lose it!" It tells you exactly how many calories to eat in a day to achieve optimal weight loss and has a calorie counter with thousands of food items to help you along your way. Losing weight is hard. The good news is that when you lose the first five pounds, you gain confidence and it gets easier.